Healing Plants of Renaissance Florence

The Development of Herbal Medicine in Florence

T0282022

Healing Plants of Renaissance Florence

The Development of Herbal Medicine in Florence

Angela Paine

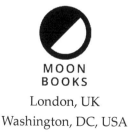

MOON
BOOKS

London, UK
Washington, DC, USA

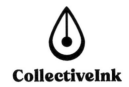

CollectiveInk

First published by Moon Books, 2024
Moon Books is an imprint of Collective Ink Ltd.,
Unit 11, Shepperton House, 89 Shepperton Road, London, N1 3DF
office@collectiveinkbooks.com
www.collectiveinkbooks.com
www.moon-books.net

For distributor details and how to order please visit the 'Ordering' section on our website.

ISBN: 978 1 80341 311 2
978 1 80341 312 9 (ebook)
Library of Congress Control Number: 2023942290

A CIP catalogue record for this book is available from the British Library.

Design: Lapiz Digital Services

UK: Printed and bound by CPI Group (UK) Ltd, Croydon, CR0 4YY
Printed in North America by CPI GPS partners

We operate a distinctive and ethical publishing philosophy in
all areas of our business, from our global network of authors to
production and worldwide distribution.

Contents

Other Books by Angela Paine

The Healing Power of Celtic Plants
Their history, their use, and the scientific evidence that they work
ISBN 978190547628

Healing Plants of the Celtic Druids
Ancient Celts in Britain and their Druid healers
used plant medicine to treat the mind body and soul
ISBN 9781785355547

Healing Plants of Greek Myth
The origins of Western medicine and its original
plant remedies derived from Greek myth
ISBN 9781789045284

Acknowledgements

Many thanks to my son, Robert Pettena, who took me to hidden places of interest in and around Florence and helped me with research for this book. And many thanks to John Daniell who helped me with the botanical drawings for the books. I'm grateful to the Santa Maria Nuova Hospital in Florence for showing me their *Orto dei Semplici* (Herb Garden) and to Emanuele Casamassima, former Director of the Bibliotecca Nazionale (National Library) in Florence for employing me after the flood in the great book restoration project which resulted in my enduring love of the city. Thank you to Sheila Barker who directed me to the Medici Archive Project. I am grateful to Cristina Bellorini, whose study of the account books of the apothecary shop, the *Speziale al Giglio*, in the archive of the *Ospedale degli Innocenti* and the Florentine Pharmacopoeia, the *Ricettariao Fiorentino,* provided me with the names of many of the plants I chose to focus on. As always, many thanks to the lovely Trevor Greenfield, who answered all my questions with remarkable speed and to all those at Moon Books who were involved in this project.

Part 1

Introduction

How I Came to Write This Book

As I stepped out of Santa Maria Novella station, Florence, into the wintery sunshine of February 1967, my feet took me into one of the dark, narrow streets of the mediaeval city. They led me between the high walls of old buildings until I came out onto the banks of the Arno, flooded with sunshine. I looked across at the narrow terracotta buildings lining the opposite river bank, church steeples rising above, the Ponte Vecchio stretching across the river on my left with all its tiny box-like shops jostling for space and I was overcome with a feeling of familiarity. I knew in that instant that I had been here in another life and determined to find a way to stay. I turned left and walked along the river bank until I came to the British Consulate, an imposing grey stone building. I entered an arch way and walked up the wide, stone steps to the front door on the first floor. An elegant English woman sitting behind a desk greeted me.

"Can I help you?"

"I'm looking for work and a place to stay," I said without preamble.

"They're hiring at the National Library," she said "and I hear the doss house in Via della Chiesa is scrubbed out with disinfectant every day."

On the 4th November 1966 Florence was hit by a devastating flood, which covered art works and hundreds of thousands of ancient books in mud, diesel and worse. I spent several months working in the National Library, where I joined an army of volunteers employed on the book restoration project, my task being to wash mud from the pages of ancient books, books I would never otherwise have had the opportunity to see, let alone touch. This led to a life-long association with the city. Time passed, I returned to England where I began to study herbalism and eventually obtained a PhD in medicinal plant chemistry.

Leonardo da Vinci

Fast forward to 2019 when, on one of my many trips to Florence, I went to a spectacular exhibition: *The Botany of Leonardo da Vinci*, at Santa Maria Novella (the convent from which the station takes its name.) The exhibition, bringing together art, nature and science, looked at the interconnections between nature and humans and celebrated the five hundredth anniversary of the death of Leonardo. It was held in the dormitory and great cloister of the Santa Maria complex, built between 1340 and 1360, where Leonardo sketched preparatory cartoons for the Battle of Anghiari in the early sixteenth century.

The first thing I saw as I entered the magnificent grand cloister, was a row of living plants in terracotta pots: sage, ivy, juniper, carob tree, strawberry tree, bamboo, box, camphor tree, two types of lemon, orange, myrtle, mastic, cork oak and bay laurel. I read that these were plants that Leonardo had drawn or written about and I realised that all but five were medicinal; and box was a herb garden hedging plant. Cork would have been used to make stoppers for jars and vials of medicinal unguents, oils and tinctures. Medicine at this time was based on the use of healing plants, so it was natural that Leonardo would have chosen these to draw.

Further along the cloister I came to a wonderful alchemical retort: a large conical vessel with a flat bottom and pointed top, whose surface was punctured by multiple round holes, from which strange bulbous structures protruded, each ending in a narrow outlet. This, I discovered, was a reproduction of one of the alchemical kilns from St Mark's convent, used for distilling plants, which would be placed inside with water, and heated from underneath. The distillate would drip from the bulbous protuberances into containers strategically placed. I read that the essential oils they produced were used to create perfumes, salves and ointments. I imagined black cloaked monks working in dark underground vaults, enveloped in swirling steam and smoke while they stirred oils and heated fats, carefully adding drops of essential oils, pouring the resultant concoctions into glass vials, stoppered with corks.

I entered the dormitory, a fabulous wonderland of plants, machines and light shows, and examined Leonardo's exquisite plant drawings. I read translations of his mirror writings, taken from the Royal Collection in Windsor Castle: 'Because nature is concerned only in the production of simple things, but man from simple things produces an infinity of compounds...' Leonardo wrote, clearly referring to individual healing plants. These at the time were known as 'simples,' whereas mixtures of these plants were known as 'compounds.' Man, he continued, 'has no power to create any simple thing...And of this the alchemists of old will bear witness, who never, by chance or planned experiment, happened to create the smallest thing which can be created by nature.' This is still true today, apart from the reference to alchemists, since plants manufacture the most complex healing compounds, which no chemist in their wildest dreams could ever create. He continues: 'This generation deserves infinite praises for the usefulness of the things which they have discovered for the use of men; and they would deserve them more if they had not been the inventors of noxious things like poisons and other similar things which destroy life or mind...' I was struck by the prescience of Leonardo's writings, even more relevant today as our health is constantly endangered by pollution from a multitude of different man-made sources.

Leonardo was alive between 1452 and 1519, during the early Renaissance, when plant medicine was used in the very few hospitals that existed. It was, however, practiced far more widely by monks in monasteries, nuns in nunneries and the general public, who probably went in search of the plants they needed in the countryside. The young Leonardo spent a considerable amount of his time between 1481–1482 producing *molti fiori ritratti al naturale* (many flowers portrayed from nature), as he wrote in his *Codex Atlanticus*. He depicted the delicate fleshiness of the petals and bracts of a Madonna lily with great skill in his drawing: *Lilium candidum* (Royal Library, Windsor Castle,) taking the trouble to draw the blossoms in various stages of flowering. He achieved an almost palpable realism through his use of chalk and wash. His pen and ink sketches of flowers of a common pear (*Pyrus communis*), the sweet violet (*Viola odorata*), a flowering stem of pearl grass (*Briza maxima*), and various species of roses are scrupulously accurate.

His fascination with nature, his understanding of sacred geometry, the meaning of Phi, the Fibonacci sequence and the Golden Ratio perhaps point to Leonardo's knowledge of Alchemy. The alchemical transmutation of base metals into gold, called the *Magnum Opus* or the *Great Work* also represented the transformation of the human soul and the achievement of enlightenment, something that Carl Jung came to understand many centuries later. Leonardo believed the workings of the human body represented the workings of the universe: As above, so below, an alchemical idea that the church did not approve of. In Leonardo's time alchemical ideas were necessarily hidden to avoid the all-seeing censor of the Roman Catholic Church, which may go some way toward explaining why Leonardo wrote in mirror writing.

He placed his drawing of Vitruvian Man inside a square and a circle as a holographic form with sixteen different positions. The square represented material existence and the circle spiritual existence, squaring the circle meaning achieving the impossible, another alchemical idea. The square unfolded revealed the tetrahedron, two joined triangles that form the

Hebrew Ker Ka Ba, meaning light, spirit, body, or light body, the energy field surrounding all living things. The spinning of the two triangles in opposing directions causes the vibration of the physical body to transform into the higher frequencies of the diamond or golden body, another alchemical idea. The exhibition was careful to avoid these ideas, though large three-dimensional representations of Leonardo's tetrahedrons were prominently displayed all over Florence.

The Santa Maria Nuova Hospital

I left the exhibition, already feeling inspired to research the plant medicine of Leonardo's time: the Renaissance. I went to visit the oldest hospital in Florence: the Santa Maria Nuova Hospital, since I had heard that it contained a herb garden. The hospital is housed in a beautiful porticoed building, whose entrance walls are adorned with colourful frescos of the Virgin Mary by Cristoforo Roncalli, 1552–1626, one of three painters known as Pomarancio. I discovered that this hospital, founded in 1288 by Folco di Ricovero dei Portinari, father of Dante's Beatrice, was still functional. The frescoes I admired were just a few of the profusion of paintings and sculptures, mostly of the Virgin Mary, by the best Renaissance Florentine artists, that once covered the internal walls.

Why, I wondered, was the Virgin Mary so venerated in Italy? The ancient hospital is named after her. Shrines to her can be found in every nook and cranny, even in the fields and forests of Italy and France. Even the central station in Florence is called Santa Maria Novella, reflecting the convent opposite of the same name, where I saw the Leonardo exhibition. The reason, I discovered, went back to the Council of Ephesus in 431 CE. Ephesus was the home of one of the seven wonders of the ancient world: the Temple of Artemis, ancient Greek virgin goddess, protector of mothers and children, probably worshipped since prehistoric times as a divine goddess and mother of the Gods.

In Ephesus debate between Christians and Artemis worshipers grew so heated that church leaders from all parts of the Christian world at that time agreed to meet there to debate the status of Mary. A vote was taken and it was decided that she was *Theotokos:* Mother of God. This did not make Mary a goddess but it did elevate her to divine. The Ephesians who had lost their goddess Artemis were appeased.

In ancient Italy, as in all Europe the goddess religion ruled for thousands of years. Italian people in Renaissance Italy still needed a divine mother figure, which the church was happy to supply in the form of the Virgin Mary. The sick in the hospital were surrounded by beautiful images of her, sometimes holding the baby Jesus. This was part of a whole system of decoration in churches and other public buildings in Florence which embodied divine action and represented the entire praying Christian community. Patients contemplating the paintings which surrounded them could absorb the healing spiritual energy generated by the prayers of the Christian community. Some might feel that the Virgin Mary was overlooking and protecting them, helping them to overcome their sickness. The pragmatic nuns who ran the hospital also grew the healing herbs they needed to treat the sick.

As I walked through the hospital entrance I saw a courtyard with terracotta pots of herbs.

"Come this way," a helpful member of staff said to me in Italian. "Step into the *Orto dei Semplici* courtyard," (herb garden for single medicinal plants,) he said.

"The original herb garden was replaced by a *Medicherie* (Medication) cloister in 1420, with a new herb garden called an *Orto dei Semplici.*"

"But this garden looks new."

"Yes over the centuries it fell into disrepair so we made a replica of it."

He left me to admire the herbs in the little courtyard.

I noticed that each herb was labelled with its common name (in Italian) and Latin binomial, together with its healing properties. There were twenty six different plants arranged symmetrically.

Some of the plants in the replica garden were chosen because monasteries and other hospitals in the area were growing them. *Sedum telephium,* (Orpine) was (and still is) grown in the Vallombrosa Abbey and the San Giovanni di Dio Hospital. Balsam was used in the ancient Santa Maria Novella perfume-pharmaceutical workshop, no longer extant but brought to life in my imagination during my visit to the Leonardo exhibition.

Other plants, such as plantain and rose, were chosen because people used them frequently. Many of the plants were part of the famous *Teriaca* composition, otherwise known as Venice treacle, composed of sixty four ingredients and said to be a cure for almost everything, including snake bite, poisoning and plague. Some plants were chosen for the part they played in electuaries prepared in the Santa Maria Nuova *spezeria* (apothecary.) Some of the most interesting plants, such as Mandrake, were chosen for their magic properties, others, such as Sage, for their religious significance. Popular plants, such as periwinkle or *Robbia,* were also included. The garden represented an entire world of medical and non-medical popular culture.

This was the first medicinal herb garden within a hospital, according to Giovanni Targioni Tozzetti, Prefect of the Florence medicinal herb garden in 1748. By the 15th century this 'simple garden' supplied herbs to the Apothecary's shop in the Hospital.

The embryo of an idea for a book of Florentine healing herbs began to form in my mind. But it was not until I discovered that the Medici family were herbal doctors, who not only made their own medicines but grew medicinal plants in herb gardens in and around Florence, that the idea for a book really began to take shape.

The Medici Family

The Renaissance, between the fourteenth and seventeenth centuries, was a period of artistic, political and economic rebirth. It was an age of exploration, from the early voyages of the Dutch, Portuguese, English and French to south east Asia; to the later Portuguese and Spanish voyages to the Caribbean and the Americas. Competition between the various nations involved in these exploratory journeys resulted in savage wars and extermination of entire civilisations. The pragmatic British Walter Raleigh sometimes saved himself the trouble of long voyages by capturing Spanish ships, laden with gold and/or spices on their return journeys. In 1592 he captured the Madre de Dios and "discovered the secret trades and Indian riches which hitherto lay strangely hidden and cunningly concealed from us." These riches included pepper, cloves, mace, nutmegs, cinnamon, ginger, benzoin, frankincense, galingale, aloes and camphor.

When Columbus set off across the Atlantic he was convinced that he would find all the spices from the East Indies in the lands he expected to find in the west: lands which came to be known as the West Indies. But he was disappointed. None were growing where he landed. So on his second journey he took spices from South East Asia to sell or exchange in the West Indies, where he found allspice, vanilla, and red peppers. In 1493 he found chilli and five capsicum species. Subsequent journeys resulted in tomatoes, cacao, haricot beans, maize, sweet potatoes, bananas and pineapples, all of which made their way to Africa, Europe and South Asia. Very few medicinal plants from the Americas made their way across the Atlantic during the Renaissance. By 1567 only guaiacum wood, china root, Western balsam (from the west indies) and sarsaparilla had been included in the *Ricettario Fiorentino* (Florentine pharmacopoeia.) American aloe and tobacco also made their way to Florence and Pisa. People thought that tobacco, kept in the mouth, strengthened the body and cured tumours and cancers and that tobacco smoke was a remedy against fatigue.

Citrus fruits from Asia were still considered exotic in Italy in the fifteenth century but Columbus took them to the Americas. Sugar cane, which originated in New Guinea, spread west to South East Asia around 3500 BCE, then to China and India in 3000 BCE. It spread slowly, reaching Europe considerably later. By the Renaissance, sugar was considered an exotic and expensive spice in Europe. The transport of plants across the world by explorers was to change the world irrevocably.

By the sixteenth century there was a ferment of discovery and innovation in the world of plants, visible in the text and illustrations of printed books, paintings, drawings and dried plant collections. Many people worked with plants during the Renaissance: herb women, midwives, folk healers, alchemists, apothecaries, monks, nuns, peasants, farmers, landowners, gardeners, traders in spices and medicines. A frisson of excitement hovered in the air as people discussed the new spices, food and medicinal plants.

At the centre of the Renaissance was Florence, with its Medici families, bankers and rulers of the city. They were finding ways to make money that did not involve plunder, murder and enslavement. Their banking systems were innovative and helpful to travelling traders, eager to avoid transporting easily stolen gold coins, and their relationship with the Pope ensured their continuing wealth. They spent the money they made lavishly on art, architectural projects, beautiful gardens and the collection of plants, especially medicinal plants. Their patronage led to new forms of plant classification, beautiful and accurate medicinal plant drawings and paintings, new ways to prepare plant medicines, new university faculties dedicated to teaching plant medicine, complete with botanical gardens for the study of the living plants. Their patronage of philosophers led to new ways of viewing life. Their patronage of alchemy led to all manner of scientific discoveries and new ways of purifying metals and plant distillation techniques.

Giovanni di Bicci

The founder of the Medici dynasty, Giovanni di Bicci (1360–1429), learned the business of banking in Rome in a distant cousin's banking house. He returned to Florence in 1397 to found his bank, subsequently creating a lucrative partnership with the Catholic Church in Rome and building up a banking system that competing bankers could not match. He tapped into foreign trade networks, providing letters of foreign exchange and establishing branches in major trading centres across Europe. This meant that traders could now carry a piece of paper representing the sum they had deposited in the city they had left and pick up the equivalent sum in the city they arrived in, paying a percentage to the bank for providing the service. Traders embraced this new safer method of transferring money across Europe and the Medici Bank flourished. Giovanni di Bicci also developed a revolutionary new double entry system for tracking deposits and withdrawals, which made it much easier to keep tabs on the financial state of the bank. He virtually invented modern banking and accountancy, over time becoming the Pope's primary banker, a lucrative and powerful position.

His family also oversaw the mining, storage and marketing of alum, an indispensable commodity for leather tanning, textile dyeing and glassmaking; as well as iron ore extraction from the island of Elba. They owned *botteghe di lana* (wool shops) and *bottege di seta* (silk shops) which farmed out the raw materials to the workers' homes and later collected the finished textiles. This system still exists in Prato, to the north of Florence, where families weave beautiful fabrics on looms in their homes. The Medici built up a huge fortune over the years.

Cosimo the Elder

Giovanni di Bicci was succeeded by Cosimo the elder (1389–1464), a successful banker and patron of the arts, learning, architecture and science. He hired Michelozzi to create the enormous, austere Palazzo Medici in Florence and commissioned him to design the first public library at San Marco. He built churches, monasteries and other buildings in and around Florence.

Under Cosimo's patronage, Florence became a centre of humanism and the most active, intellectual and artistic centre in Europe. He was never a ruler of Florence, but kept a close eye on the affairs of the city, befriending Poggio Bracciolini, the chancellor, historian, moralist and scholar of classical antiquities, who also recovered many classical texts. Cosimo was so enamoured of Greek learning that he supported a group of philosophers: Poliziano, Cristofero Landino, Pico della Mirandola and the brilliant polymath and humanist philosopher, Marsilio Ficino, (1433–99.)

In 1453, during a voyage to Macedonia Leonardo of Pistoia discovered fourteen books supposedly written by Hermes Trismegistus in the eleventh century: the *Hermetica*. Hermes Trismegistus (Hermes thrice great) was a fusion of the Greek Hermes, god of communication, and the Egyptian god of letters, Thoth. Leonardo brought them back to Florence and gave them to Cosimo, who asked Ficino to translate the Greek into Latin in 1463. Ficino called his translation Pimander and it became a great success, translated into many languages. The influence of the mythical Hermes Trismegistus, spread far and wide, adopted as a real Egyptian sage by the alchemists, as a contemporary of Moses by the Cabalists and discussed endlessly by Renaissance philosophers.

Ficino immersed himself in the fourteen books that comprised the Hermetica, absorbing their philosophy, which claimed that the Heavens had equal counterparts on Earth, and vice versa. He took this pre-Christian idea and connected it to the Christian concept of the human soul, which he was convinced linked the world of the intellect with that of nature. He believed souls were immortal and the soul's vehicles transported its memories through the universe, keeping them alive, a foreshadowing of Jung's collective consciousness.

He suggested that the soul had more than one vehicle. One, the air vehicle, the *spiritus*, based in the brain, was responsible for perception, imagination and memory. Another, the ethereal vehicle, existed before the earthly body came into being and survived after death. He believed that the power of imagination was stronger than that of the four senses and that the soul was more intensely perceptive after death.

Ficino found many connections between the Hermetica and the philosophies of Plato, which up until this time had not been translated. Most people's knowledge of Plato's philosophy was largely indirect and incomplete, and both Cosimo and Ficino were convinced that a complete translation was essential for the development of Humanism. So Cosimo gave Ficino a house in Fiesole, and the income from a rental property and in 1462 he commissioned him to translate the entire works of Plato into Latin and to found an *Accademia Platónica*: Platonic Academy, together with Poliziano, Cristofero Landino and Pico della Mirandola. In 1464, Ficino read his translations of Plato's dialogues to Cosimo as the ageing patron lay dying. Ficino, who identified Plato's theory of love with Christian love, invented the phrase Platonic love. His translation was not published until 1484, but went through many editions and profoundly influenced philosophy and humanism.

Cosimo was patron of Fra Angelico, Fra Filippo Lippi and Donatello, as well as the architect Brunelleschi, who created the fabulous dome of the Florence Duomo (the cathedral) in 1436. He financed the painter, Pontormo, who worked at his court for many years, where he painted his portrait with a laurel plant beside him, among whose leaves is entwined a scroll with a verse from Virgil that alludes to the regeneration, like a vigorous plant, of the Medici stock: *Uno anulso non déficit alter.* (When the first is torn away, a second does not fail.) He was an amateur alchemist and the lengths he went to in order to acquire a 13th-century manuscript of Pliny's Natural History, indicate his interest in plant medicine, according to Sheila Barker.

He provided his grandson, Lorenzo de' Medici, with a humanist education that covered classical literature, history, rhetoric, dialectic, natural philosophy, arithmetic, Greek and modern foreign languages. His tutors were the diplomat and bishop Gentile de Becchi and Marsilio Ficino. He taught Lorenzo's brother, Giuliano, the principles of banking.

Lorenzo the Magnificent

Cosimo's son Piero died two years after his father, leaving Cosimo's grandsons, Lorenzo (1449–1492) and Giuliano (1453–1478) in control of the bank. The two young men were ill-prepared for this daunting task and at the mercy of another banking family, the Pazzi, who were in cahoots with the Archbishop of Pisa and several other important people who were conspiring to overthrow them. On Sunday 26 April 1478 the plotters attacked the brothers in the cathedral of Florence, killing Giuliano. The people of Florence rallied round Lorenzo, defending him from his enemies. They supported him. They loved him, calling him *Il Magnifico*: the Magnificent. He was now the sole male adult survivor of the family, heir to the fortune his grandfather had amassed.

Lorenzo ushered in a period of peace and tranquility, winning the hearts and minds of the people, but unfortunately the Pope had ceased to have financial dealings with him, so this important source of revenue had been cut off. But this was of no interest to the people of Florence, used as they were to the generous Medici family, who appeared to have bottomless coffers of gold coins which they dispensed in payment for all manner of projects.

Lorenzo was interested in everything: art, science, botany, medicine and he encouraged stimulating interchanges between the different disciplines. Artists, architects and philosophers were drawn to Florence by news of his generosity and Lorenzo responded by surrounding himself with artists, such as Sandro Botticelli, Andrea del Verocchio and Verocchio's pupil, Leonardo da Vinci, treating them affectionately and commissioning them to paint the beautiful masterpieces that continue to enrapture visitors to Florence. He opened a school of sculpture in his garden near the church of San Marco and it was there that he met the already brilliant fifteen year old Michelangelo. He spent a fortune on ancient texts and may have instigated the first Florentine Pharmacopeia, according to Paolo Galluzzi in 1980. He was deeply interested in medicine and collected ancient Greek treatises on surgery.

He patronised architects, writers and philosophers and continued to finance Marsillio Ficino's Platonic Academy. This created a cultural ambience in Florence rarely matched elsewhere for its dynamism.

By the mid-1470s interest in ancient texts such as Pliny the Elder's *Historia Naturalis* led to artists paying greater attention to the detail of the plants they were depicting. Lorenzo, and other members of the Medici dynasty, sponsored botanical art, resulting in the creation of numerous paintings of plants, both medicinal and decorative. During this period artists who flocked to Florence, drawn by the promise of funds that would enable them to paint, produced works of artistic quality, refinement, and sophisticated ideological content that would never be surpassed. They developed a complex symbology, full of plant references, often painting meadows of flowers.

One of the most famous examples of a flowering meadow is Botticelli's *Primavera* (Spring) now in the Uffizi Gallery,

Florence. Botticelli, who recognised all the flowers that grew around Florence in the different seasons, knew that Lorenzo would notice the plants in his paintings so his depictions of these flowers was meticulously accurate in every detail, including the time of their flowering:

between April and May. The only exceptions were the hellebore, which blooms in January, and the coltsfoot (*Tussilago farfara*), which flowers in March. Unfortunately on May 18th, 1492, Lorenzo died from an inherited autoimmune disease, probably acromegaly, according to Lippi in 2017.

Lorenzo's son Piero was twenty when his father died in 1492. He became the next ruler of Florence, only to discover that his father had virtually bankrupted the family. Lacking his father's diplomatic skills, he made a terrible mess of ruling Tuscany, the Florentines attacked and ransacked his palace and he and his brothers fled.

Savonarola, the fanatical puritan friar, became the moral dictator of Florence. But his rule was short. By 1498 the Florentine authorities had arrested him, condemned him as a heretic, hung him and burnt him at the stake. In 1512 Giovanni de' Medici, the cardinal, persuaded the Pope to restore the Medici to Florence, a year before he became Pope Leo X. In 1527 the Medici were thrown out of Florence again. In 1532 a new constitution established Alessandro de' Medici as the hereditary Duke of Florence.

Cosimo I de' Medici

In 1537 at the tender age of seventeen, Cosimo I de' Medici (1519–1574) inherited the title of Grand Duke of Florence from his cousin, Alessandro, who was assassinated after a mere five years in power. He was well-liked and became known as *Cosimo il Grande*: Cosimo the Great. In 1539 he married Eleonora of Toledo, which helped to cement a Medici alliance with Spain. In 1540 they moved from the Palazzo Medici in via Larga to

Palazzo Vecchio, until then the seat of the Florentine Republic. He chose the brilliant artist, architect, engineer, writer and historian, Giorgio Vasari, to be his superintendent of buildings and commissioned him to redecorate the interior of Palazzo Vecchio. He then set about bringing almost all of Tuscany under his control through a series of military battles and clever diplomacy. Once he had pacified his potential enemies, he brought the state administration under his control by uniting all the public services in a single building: the Uffizi (Offices) which he commissioned Vasari to design.

In 1549 his wife, Eleonora, bought the Pitti Palace. Cosimo immediately asked Vasari to enlarge the building and to build the secret passageway above the shops that line the Ponte Vecchio, a passageway that still to this day links the Uffizi with the Pitti Palace. In view of the recent assassination of his cousin, Alessandro, the earlier assassination of his great uncle, Giuliano, and the attempt on Lorenzo's life, it's understandable that Cosimo would want to protect his family and himself from potential assassins. These were dangerous times.

When Eleonora bought the Pitti Palace the hill behind it was a rough wilderness covering a hundred and eleven acres. In 1550 when she and Cosimo moved into the palace, she commissioned the architect, Nicolò Tribolo, to design a garden. This was a serious challenge, not only due to the hilly terrain but also because there was no water supply. Unfortunately Tribolo died later that year but Bartolomeo Ammanati continued the work. Eleonora took an interest in the layout and iconography of the gardens but left the choice of plants to Cosimo. Vasari helped with the planning and Bernardo Buontalenti contributed sculptures. They had to design a conduit to bring water from the Arno River to the gardens to water the newly planted trees and hedges and feed the fountains, grottoes and other water features. It became known as the Boboli Garden, the private garden of the Medici family and their friends. Agostino Lapini in his Florentine Journal said:

> On Monday 12 May 1550 we started to level the ground in the garden at Pitti and provide it with drains, to plant firs, cypresses, ilexes and bays.

Nowadays we are used to seeing these plants in Tuscany but maybe they were not so common in the sixteenth century.

Cosimo's name, like that of his forebears, underlined his medical practice, for *Medici* is the plural of *medico*, Italian for doctor, and the name Cosimo reflects *Cosmas*, one of the two patron saints of physicians and apothecaries. He came from a long line of medicinal plant enthusiasts. Caterina Sforza, his grandmother, left him three volumes of pharmaceutical secrets while his mother busied herself concocting herbal potions, such as the one she used to deworm his children, according to Barker in 2016. His predecessor Alessandro de' Medici was a medical reformer who helped to establish the Florence Hospital for the incurable sufferers of the French Pox (syphilis.) Cosimo was passionately interested in plant medicine. Vincenzo Fedeli felt that he excelled in botany above all his other accomplishments, which were many.

Cosimo was so excited by the ancient world of plant medicine that he determined to promote it in every way. He commissioned Pietro Andrea Mattioli to translate Dioscorides' *de Materia Medica* into Italian. Mattioli began his translation in 1541, accompanying each entry with a rich commentary on the identification of the specimen. At that time botanical illustrations in Italy were completely useless, since they were copied from other drawings and in no way resembled the plants they were supposed to represent, so there were no drawings in the original edition.

The first really accurate plant illustrations had already appeared in Germany by the founders of botany: Otto Brunfels (1488–1534), Leonhart Fuchs (1501–1566), and Hieronymus Bock (1498–1554.) Brunfels was the first to write a herbal, *Herbarum Vivae Eicones,* with accurate botanical illustrations by Hans Weiditz, between 1530 and 1536. Fuchs published *De Historia Stirpium* in Latin in 1542, an absolutely enormous book with the most accurate woodcut illustrations of plants yet published. It took Fuchs thirty years to complete this, his greatest work. He asked his artists to depict ideal plants, with no imperfections, and to show all a plant's blooming process, including flowers and seeds. The overall accuracy of the illustrations was remarkable and the images are very useful for the identification of the plants. The technique he asked his artists to adopt, that of drawing only the outlines of the plants, has become the standard botanical drawing technique still used today. He employed the artist, Albrecht Meyer to paint the plants, the copyist Heinrich Fullmaurer to make drawings, and Veit Rudolf Speckle, the unrivalled master, to make the engravings from the drawings. In the preface to his work, Fuchs explained that this book was for the benefit of his fellow physicians, who, he stated had no accurate knowledge of the plants they used as medicine.

Mattioli's book, *I Discorsi di M Pietro Andrea Matthioli...nei sei Libri di Pedacio Dioscoride Anazarbeo Della Materia Medicinale,* published in Venice in 1544, was a huge success. By 1554, by which time people had become aware of the wonderful German herbals, the *Discorsi* was republished with five hundred woodcuts of the plants. In 1562 a Prague publisher commissioned new larger woodcuts by Giorgio Liberale and Wolfgang Meyerpeck for another edition. These woodcuts were superbly detailed. Mattioli described more plants and gathered information from his colleagues which he incorporated into his ever-extending commentaries in each new edition. Paula Findlen sees the

Discorsi as a centre around which a natural history community began to form. It became the best-selling scientific book of the Renaissance, the various versions selling 32,000 copies, possibly because the woodcuts were so beautiful.

By 1543 Cosimo had read, learned and absorbed Dioscorides' *de Materia Medica* in the original Greek and was using it as a reference book for the identification of plants. He went through the first edition of Mattioli's *Discorsi*, making notes in the margins, and since he didn't agree with all his (Mattioli's) vernacular plant names, he sponsored a new translation into the Florentine language by Marcantonio Montesiano in 1545. The medical doctor, Baccio Baldini said of Cosimo:

[He] knew of a great quantity of plants; he knew where they grow, where they thrive longest, where they produce the largest harvests, where they render the most flavourful fruits, the times when they flower and fructify, and the benefits of these plants, many of which can cure the diseases of both humans and animals.

Filippo Pigafetta said that Cosimo's *fonderia* (alchemical laboratory) was a place:

...where they continuously distil waters of scented flowers and herbs, and oils from drugs and spices producing quintessence and ointments and make electuaries and curative confections, liquors for malignant fevers, plague, and poisons, and powders, and medicines of powerful and prompt virtues.

Cosimo sent people far and wide on book finding expeditions and bought Leonhart Fuchs's fabulously expensive *Herbarum ac stirpium historia*. Even though Cosimo preferred to observe living plants, the accuracy of the illustrations in Fuchs's book inspired him to encourage the artists he patronised to paint plants in as much lifelike detail as possible.

Vasari noted that the duke loved pharmaceutical plants so much that in 1545 he commissioned Francesco Ubertini (known as Bachiacca) to paint life size images of them on the walls of his private study in Palazzo Vecchio, the same year that he commissioned the new translation of Dioscorides' *de Materia Medica*. Cosimo instructed him to paint the plants from living specimens wherever possible and to use the dried, flattened specimens from the expert botanist, Luca Ghini's herbarium if the living specimens were not available. Bachiacca's paintings of Tuscan wild or medicinal plants were meticulously accurate in every detail, even showing the root systems, to facilitate correct identification. Cosimo, impressed by Fuchs' *Herbarum ac stirpium historia,* wanted Bachiacca to paint the plants as accurately as those in Fuchs' herbal. Benedetto Varchi noted that the botanical murals in Cosimo's study were of "very great utility for the sciences." Giovanni Targioni Tozzetti suggested that Cosimo wanted these paintings on the walls of his study and living plants in his botanical gardens "to impress their appearances deeply into the memory."

Cosimo wanted all the plants that were used in ancient Greek medicine for his various herb gardens, but this was becoming increasingly difficult due to more and more piracy in the Mediterranean and the heating up of religious wars, according to Barker in 2015. The *Ricettario Fiorentino* explained:

With regard to the herbs that were prized in antiquity, produced in certain places where today it is no longer possible to travel, it is necessary to make every effort to search for similar ones in our lands and to see whether they have the same benefits as the former.

He decided to grow as many of the ancient Greek medicinal plants as possible.

The Studio Pisano (University of Pisa) was founded in 1343, and from 1473, when Lorenzo the Magnificent moved the state's university from Florence to Pisa, it became the principal university of Tuscany. Unfortunately Pisa and Florence were at loggerheads in the early sixteenth century and the Studio had to shut its doors. Cosimo reopened it in 1543. He wanted to restore it to its former level of academic excellence. He immediately set up a college to care for poor students in order to provide for those who 'oppressed by domestic poverty could not, without such help, show the excellence and nobility of their minds.' He sponsored the first botany professorship, setting up a chair of 'Simple Medicaments.'

He made generous offers to celebrated scientists from all over Europe, including Leonhart Fuchs, who refused his offer. Distinguished physicians, such as Matteo Corti, Leonardo Giacchino, Giovanni Argenterio accepted Cosimo's invitation. Luca Ghini, the brilliant botanist, was lecturing in the university of Bologna when Cosimo invited him to come to Pisa. He agreed to leave Bologna on condition that he be allowed to create a botanic garden where he could grow plants from seed, transplant and propagate them, examine and monitor their development and use them to teach his students to recognise the plants they would use as medicine. He pointed out that theoretical knowledge was not much use unless the students could study living plant specimens.

Before Ghini arrived in Pisa the study of medicine was theoretical, the plant medicines that doctors prescribed being made up by apothecaries, who bought the plants from the peasants and old women who recognised and collected them, while the doctors who used them knew little about them. The peasants' knowledge was passed down orally from generation to generation. So Ghini's suggestion that students of medicine should actually study the plants they would use to treat their patients was revolutionary.

Cosimo supported Ghini wholeheartedly and agreed to finance Europe's first botanical garden in Pisa, which Ghini created between the years 1543 and 1544. He was Cosimo's personal physician, had a profound influence on him, and shared his enthusiasm for living, healing plants. They both wanted the botanic garden to be like a living book, containing every species mentioned in the ancient pharmaceutical herbals.

Ghini and his assistants went on plant collecting expeditions for the botanic garden. He sent out requests to colleagues and correspondents, who sent him specimens. He planted 620 medicinal herbs, according to Aldrovandi, who made a list, the first list of plant seeds in the history of botany. Botanists were permitted to use the seeds produced by the herbs in the botanic garden, and this resulted in a web of correspondence, exchanges and requests. Greene spoke about Ghini's tendency to joke about Dioscorides:

...the very etymology of the name Dioscorides shows what kind of man he was; that Greek name always sounded to him like *Deus Discordiae*. And really what the good old man said in jest and to provoke a laugh is not far from being true. Dioscorides did indeed transmit so great a number of succinct, short, shabby and imperfect plant descriptions that, through such brief hints as he has given it may be impossible to arrive at a determination of the plants; hence concerning many of them we have such a variety of opinions, such seemingly opposite judgements about so many plants as renders it doubtful whether they can be recognised if ever found...

Benedetto Varchi said of Ghini:

And though the custom of modern philosophers is always to believe what is written in the classical authors and most of all in Aristotle, without proving anything, sometimes it is no less a sure thing to do otherwise and to depend on *experienza* (personal observation); I found some others who share this opinion, especially Luca Ghini, most distinguished physician and herbalist.

Despite his scepticism, Ghini based his research on Dioscorides' work, always checking and reorganising, comparing the botanical text with the living plants, seeking them out, drawing and commissioning artists to paint pictures of them, growing and recording them in his herbarium. Seybold wrote that Ghini even sent a series of botanical illustrations to Leonhart Fuchs, who included them in his unpublished *Erbario figuarativo*, which indicates their excellence and accuracy. He drew attention to the confusion of nomenclature and the difficulty of interpretation in the field of medical botany, always trying to clarify the identity of the lesser known plants. When he was reading from Dioscorides, he took his students out into the botanical garden and pointed to the plant he was talking about.

Cosimo sent Ghini to look for the medicinal plants mentioned in ancient Greek texts, in Tuscany, telling him that when he failed to find one of these plants growing locally, he should suggest a similar substitute. He also asked him to make a note of any lost and forgotten plants people were still using as medicine. Ghini combed the Tuscan countryside and spoke to monks, merchants, seamen, soldiers, cardinals and many others who provided him with information. Whenever people gave him seeds he planted them in the botanic garden to see whether they would grow in the Tuscan soil and climate and to show them to his students if they did.

Ghini was interested in food plants as well as medicinal ones and went in search of as many exotic plants as he could, such as sunflower, maize, various types of pumpkin, and prickly pear, all from South America, and planted them in Pisa's botanic garden. He almost certainly tried to grow more plants in Pisa than those we know about. Letters of the time are full of accounts of plants which arrived in very poor condition or could not survive in the Tuscan soil and climate. Andrés Laguna, the Spanish botanist, visited the Pisa botanic garden in 1549 and said:

> All these plants I saw in Pisa, in the garden of the duke, Cosimo de' Medici, just as they are depicted by Dioscorides.

Cosimo sought out rare and interesting plants, including exotic ones from far afield, such as the Indian Banyan tree, *Ficus Benghalensis*. He asked diplomats and couriers to bring him the plants that Ghini had collected in far off places so that he could cultivate them in the gardens of his villas, including Villa Castello and the Boboli Garden.

Keen to understand the workings of the human body, Cosimo bought Vesalius's illustrated anatomy books in 1543. After reading them, he decided the study of medicine had to include anatomy so, according to Giovanni Pratilli, in 1975, he set up an anatomy chair in the faculty of Medicine in Pisa University.

Cosimo's interests ranged far and wide. Suzanne Butters shows how he was equally interested in botany, alchemy, medicine and metallurgy as well as funding numerous architectural and artistic projects in and around Florence and collecting a library of rare books in Greek and Latin. He took an interest in agriculture, and listened to the Tuscan aristocrats who provided him with information about fertiliser, planting and harvesting according to the phases of the moon, testing the soil to detect sulphur, iron, vitriol, alum and other substances that could influence the flavour of the crops. Giovanni Battista Tedaldi gave the duke the *Discorso dell'Agricultura* in 1572 which Cosimo read and made notes on. Pietro Vettori said:

(Cosimo) does not in any way scorn the cultivation of the land, nor see it as a squalid thing unworthy of (his) station to handle the plants with (his) hands on occasion and to take great care that they are well placed and that each is arranged with respect to the others.

Cosimo believed that astronomy was relevant to farming, shipbuilding and tides so he had a large astrolabe built so that he could chart the movements of the planets and stars, but he did not believe in elective astrology. He took a great interest in military engineering, important in an age of wars, though he was the first to state that "measurements and books don't fight." He needed minerals such as saltpetre, sulphur, iron, lead, copper and lime, to produce munitions, and he needed experts to identify, locate, mine and purify them. He brought back experts from Germany in 1546 to work in his mines near Pietrasanta, Massa and Campiglia and he investigated the best way to process silver ore so as to retain as much lead as possible.

Cosimo's Interest in Alchemy

What was alchemy and why was Cosimo so interested in it? Superficially it was the search for the philosopher's stone, that would transmute lesser metals into gold and was also a panacea and provider of eternal life. In fact alchemy was far more complex and intriguing. It was an interweaving of philosophical, psychological and chemical ideas, clothed in obscure symbolism that rendered it incomprehensible to all but the initiated. Its goals were both practical (better medicine and better methods of purifying metals) and esoteric (creating the philosopher's stone.) To a man like Cosimo, highly educated and interested in every aspect of life, alchemy held a deep fascination. He built a *fonderia*: a chemical-pharmaceutical, alchemical laboratory, in Palazzo Vecchio, when he was living there from 1540 to 1550, and provided funds for the most able alchemists to carry out their experiments.

Many different authors, including Michel Plaisance in 1974, mention his interest in alchemy, which possibly began when he brought samples from his mines and began experimenting in metallurgical alchemy. This provided him with useful methods for purifying the metals from his mines. Or maybe it was his passion for herbal medicine which drove him to seek better distillation methods. But by the 1550s he and his workers were involved in a great, messy, dirty melting pot of experimentation on plants and metals in his alchemical *fonderia.*

The best alchemists were not mystical dreamers, but skilled bench chemists. Several people, mentioned in the Magliabechiano XV, could have helped Cosimo, such as Cipriano Ferrini, a distiller, and Agostino Pini, who showed Cosimo how to extract silver from copper. Riguccio Galluzzi was scathing about Cosimo's passion for alchemy, which he called: "the most vain of all," and depicts Cosimo in his laboratory, taking delight in transmuting metals and producing potent poisons. However, he admits grudgingly that, "since errors and vanities sometimes lead to the discovery of useful things, this laboratory became famous all over Europe for the remedies and medicines that were there produced."

Bartolomeo Concini speaks of how Cosimo became sufficiently expert in alchemy to have perfected a method for tinting metals red. Vincenzo Fedeli reported in 1556 that: "Cosimo goes often (to his distillation laboratory) and there he works with his hands with great delight ... to discover the miracles and the secrets of nature, which mostly regard the investigation of metals."

Cosimo also read books on alchemy, such as Pompeo Florido's transcription of Christophorus Parisiensis, *L'Aspertorio Alfabeticale.* As with all the other books he read, he made copious notes in the margins.

There was an explosion of interest in distillation in the sixteenth century. Everyone who could afford to was doing it secretly, from apothecaries to people in private homes to large scale laboratories. This may have been because glass was more available, better furnaces had been invented or because there were now several distillation manuals in circulation.

Alchemical distillation had been around for several centuries, first recorded by John of Roquetaillade, known as Rupescissa, 1310–1366, a Franciscan friar from Salerno monastery.

Many alchemists joined monastic orders, according to Chiara Crisciani in 1996. Monasteries were quiet, peaceful, safe and the monks had plenty of time to carry out long, complex alchemical experiments. They could translate ancient Greek and Arabic texts into Latin. Intertwining philosophy with experimentation, Rupescissa took Aristotle's idea of an unattainable fixed essence and proposed producing it through a thousand-fold distillation of wine. This, he said, would provide a universal medicine, a *quintessenzia,* an *aqua ardens,* a panacea.

Ficino, who thought of himself as a doctor both of bodies and of souls, took Rupescissa's idea of a healing quintessence and incorporated it into his philosophy as *Spiritus Mundi*, an active component of the world soul. This was not just a philosophical idea; like Rupescissa, Ficino, who was an alchemist, in addition to philosopher, doctor of medicine and priest, attempted to create his quintessence through distillation. His philosophy, a marriage of alchemical, Platonic and Christian ideas, had a huge influence on the thought patterns of his contemporaries as well as feeding back into the symbolism of alchemy.

The involvement of monks and nuns in alchemy may explain why many alchemical writings included all kinds of religious concepts, such as comparing metals to biblical people or events. Alchemists even gave their equipment names that reflected Christian ideas: for example, the word crucible, a vessel that can withstand high heat, derives from the Latin *cruciare*: to crucify, according to Theodore Ziolkowski in 2015.

Cosimo advertised the fact that he distilled plants for medicine, but kept quiet about the alchemical experiments he and his artisans were carrying out, for alchemy was necessarily cloaked in secret symbols, hidden in complex word and picture allegories. Alchemists used cover names to hide the ingredients of their recipes. All seven metals known at the time had astrological pseudonyms: the Sun represented gold, the Moon: silver, Mercury was mercury, Venus: copper, Mars: iron, Jupiter: tin and Saturn: lead. Sometimes alchemists compared metals to pagan deities or myths. Eggs, dragons and the Phoenix referred to marriage, death and resurrection.

Despite the necessary secrecy, Florence became one of the first great centres of alchemy in Europe under Cosimo's sponsorship. Other European centres, such as Prague, under Rudolf II (1552–1612) followed his example, according to Ursula Klein.

When he and his family moved to the Pitti Palace in 1550, he had another *fonderia* built behind the palace, where the Boboli Gardens were being created, and one between the end of the Uffizi Gallery and the beginning of the corridor towards the river Arno, comprising eight rooms and a terrace. They contained alembics and glass vessels of every shape, furnaces, chimneys and numerous distillation tools and instruments. Cinelli describes two huge *circulatori magni*: furnaces with a quadruple ascending line of twelve tin flasks each penetrating the next and a similar one descending, in one of the rooms.

Artists typically painted or drew alchemists surrounded by strange vessels and dense smoke, chaos and madness, often in dilapidated buildings, with stuffed animals, such as lizards, crows or owls hanging from the rafters. The chaos and dense smoke may well have reflected aspects of Cosimo's *fonderie*, but the buildings that housed them were certainly not dilapidated and I doubt whether there were any stuffed animals or birds hanging from the ceilings.

Basic alchemical equipment included a fireplace or furnace, bellows to raise the temperature and distillation apparatus, such as an alembic. This consisted of a cucurbit: a gourd-shaped container which contained the liquid to be distilled and a cap which fitted over the mouth of the cucurbit to receive the steam, with a long sloping beak down which trickled the condensed steam into a receiving container. The alchemists' retort was a distilling vessel in which the cap and the cucurbit had been combined to form a single vessel. The retorts I saw at the Leonardo exhibition in Florence were enormous with multiple beaks projecting from their sides, veritable distillation factories.

Interestingly some of the equipment we were using to extract compounds from medicinal plants at the School of Pharmacy in London was similar to that of the alchemists. We did, however, use bunsen burners rather than fireplaces and bellows, and we did not have alchemical retorts, but the rest of our equipment differed little from that of the alchemists. They used glass beakers, flasks, crystallising dishes, funnels, filtering vessels and mortars, all of which we were also using. There was definitely less smoke in our laboratory than in that of the ancient alchemists, but almost as much chaos, at least on our benches, which were cluttered with every sort and kind of glass equipment. Of course, we had access to certain modern equipment, such as silica gel plates for separating compounds from raw plant material, a technique the alchemists would have envied, and we were able to subject the results of our work to spectroscopic analysis, something as incomprehensible to a lay person today as an alchemical formula.

Some alchemists focussed on the philosophical/psychological aspects of alchemy, seeking to perfect matter while perfecting their own inner natures. They may have followed a seven stage process:

1. Calcination: the stage in which the *materia prima* or starting material was heated so that it would produce white ashes, called a "salt" by alchemists. This was called the *albedo* (the white) stage. The root of the word calcination refers to the removal of carbon from limestone (calcium carbonate) to yield calcium oxide (quicklime). But the alchemists used the term to describe heating any starting material, such as mercury and sulphur, that could be separated by applying heat. Spiritually this represented freeing oneself from worldly attachments.

2. Dissolution, dissolving the ashes in water. During this stage one descended into the unconscious.

3. Separation, in which the pure essence was extracted from the rest of the mixture. During this stage one left the ego behind.

4. Conjunction, in which the elements were re-combined so that, by the destructive power of Mercury, the matter was gradually broken down and brought into solution.

5. Putrefaction, or fermentation, which represented 'The First Death', the first cleansing of the base matter, during which it underwent 'Mortification and Putrefaction'. This stage ended in a return to chaos which was symbolised by a blackness that alchemists called the *nigredo*. During this stage one came face to face with one's fears.

6. Distillation, in which impurities were removed. During this stage one overcame one's fears.

7. Coagulation in which the distillate was left to solidify. Spiritually this stage involved unification of spirit and matter, body and soul, masculine and feminine to form a single whole. It was called the *rubedo,* the final red stage, when the initiate became illuminated with the ultimate truth.

There were several other possible stages, such as exaltation, which referred to refining specific metals or refining the spirit of man. Multiplication was the process used to increase the potency of the philosopher's stone or elixir, towards the end of the Great Work. Cosimo may well have followed some or all of these stages in the refinement of his metals.

The church did not approve of alchemy. Nor did Dante, who put alchemists in the tenth and final pouch of the *Malebolge* (Evil Pouches) in the Eighth Circle of Hell. Cosimo's *fonderie* would indeed have resembled one of the layers of Dante's Inferno, with workers enveloped in smoke, coughing from acrid fumes as they stooped to tend the furnaces. Unafraid of these terrible conditions, Cosimo stepped into his *fonderie* to use the equipment to extract the pure virtues (quintessences) from herbs, roots, seeds, gums and minerals. But considering the multiplicity of his other interests, I doubt that he spent a great deal of time there.

Perifano noted that while he was experimenting with metals, Cosimo was also creating herbal remedies for the good of his friends and family. He may well have learned from Luca Ghini, who was expert at distilling medicinal plants and whose herbal formulas were recorded by Giovanni Battista Nardi. Baccio Baldini said:

Cosimo began to employ his knowledge of plants for the welfare and benefit of society and thus he had many kinds of plants, leaves, and flowers distilled with various methods throughout the year in order to obtain precious essences and oils; he also produced many different medicines, both simple and compound, which he gave away to any of his subjects who needed them and to individuals throughout Europe who sent him their requests.

His *spezeria* (pharmacy) was famous and its medicines much in demand. On one day in 1565 Emperor Maximilian II requested a nerve ointment, Francesco de' Medici asked for a poison antidote and Cardinal Giovanni Ricci wanted a medicine for sciatica and arthritis, according to Sheila Barker. Even the King of Spain relied on Cosimo's medications whose secret composition couldn't be replicated.

Cristina Bellorini explains that the Grand Dukes sometimes ordered their supply of healing plants from the apothecary shops, to be collected by the master of the *fonderia*. At other times they sent people to buy them in Venice, directly shipped from Spain and Portugal. They also ordered them from *erboli* or *erboristi* (herbalists) who collected them in the wild, as we can see from Niccolò Sisti's letter of 1601:

> We will give, on behalf of Vostra Signoria, lire sixteen to the herbalists Francesco di Antonio Macherini and Marco di Simone for the payment of all the herbs and roots that go into the compound of '*aqua da pietra*' and for all the herbs and other things that go into the '*olio da spasimo*', and for all the herbs and other things that go into the compound of '*olio da ferite*,' provided from the above mentioned up to this day...

Cosimo commissioned a book to record all his herbal recipes called *Book in which will be written experiments and reliable things [made] by the hand of the duke of Florence, or otherwise in his presence, nor will there be anything that is not absolutely proven for the common good*. Published in 1556, the manuscript resides in the Florence National Library and contains hundreds of recipes, such as the ones for an *elixir vitae*, a painkilling oil, a balm, a dried botanical resin oil and a poison-antidote oil. (This contained equal parts olive oil and ground up scorpions, small quantities of several herbal ingredients such as rhubarb, *Aloe patico*, lavender, saffron, catesbian gentian, tormentil, white dittany, and bistort; plus small amounts of two exceedingly expensive pharmaceutical preparations: *theriac* and *mithridate*.) The *elixir vitae* contained seventy-five ingredients. Cosimo's recipes reflect his desire to recreate the ancient Greek and Roman *materia medica*, which tended to contain multiple ingredients.

In 2015 Marinozzi explained how the duke tested his poison antidote on a criminal waiting for capital punishment. Unfortunately it did not work but this did not stop people believing that it did. Many of the ingredients in the ancient recipes came from Greece or even further afield and were rare and precious, such as dittany from Crete and cinnamon from Sri Lanka, but Cosimo sought them out, sending his agents to Venice to buy them from the newly arrived ships.

He was critical of the commercial pharmacy of his times, stating that herbal ingredients should not be boiled since the healing properties would escape with the steam, but should rather be distilled. In the case of aromatic plants he had a valid point, but he was unaware that plants rich in water-soluble compounds would have been better boiled than distilled. He also stated that pharmacists should only use glass containers for cooking the herbs, since glass was the only material that would not contaminate them. He was absolutely correct in this instance and way ahead of his time.

He replaced the old 1498 *Ricettaria fiorentino* with a new one in 1550 which included regulations for pharmacists, an alphabetical list of *materia medica,* recipes, tables of measurements and a list of possible substitutes. He instituted a college of Physicians' officers responsible for inspecting all the licensed pharmacists every year, to make sure that they complied with his regulations, according to Lucia Sandri in 2012. He also reformed the medical profession, cracking down on charlatans, unsafe procedures and fraudulent labelling. Baccio Baldini commented that an ideal prince uses his knowledge of medicine to protect his subjects from causes of disease and bodily harm and Cosimo almost certainly believed this.

The ill went to the Medici *spezeria* (pharmacy) for medicines, mine owners for better acids to dissolve ores, and painters for pigments. The preparation of pigments for artists had been perfected as far back as the fourteenth century. Cennino Cennini, a Florentine craftsman, said that vermilion pigment, made by heating mercury and sulphur together, "is made by alchemy, prepared in a retort", and was available to buy from apothecaries. It was hugely important to both alchemists and artists since it signified the final stage of the Great Work or the Red King. Daniel Thompson says "no other scientific invention has had so great and lasting an effect upon painting practice as the invention of this colour."

Renaissance artists often chose the colours they used for their symbolic and mystical meanings. Art, alchemy and colour were inextricably intertwined, since different colours signified the progress of the Great Work of the alchemists, which comprised a sequence of colour changes from white to black to yellow, ending with red. Alchemical recipes often included lead, arsenic and antimony, since some of the compounds containing these elements are these colours. Artists had long known that lead carbonate was white, lead tetroxide was red and lead monoxide was yellow, they knew arsenic sulphide could be yellow or orange, and mercury sulphide was vermillion. Cennini explains that these pigments were created by alchemists or apothecaries using alchemical ideas.

It was not only the church that wanted to eliminate the alchemists. The sovereign state used gold and silver as currency and the alchemists' attempt to transform lead into gold threatened the economic stability of the state. One of the alchemists' crafty techniques was to dip debased coins into a tincture that would make them look like gold, according to Mary Merrifield in 1849. The church condemned alchemists outright for claiming to have power over nature, since transmuting matter should be reserved for God alone, as well as for counterfeiting money. So alchemists sought wealthy patrons, such as the Medici, who would protect them from the church and state. Others, unable to enter monasteries, went into hiding.

There was one alchemist, Paracelsus (1493–1541) whose good reputation allowed him to be completely open about his practice. He let it be known that his alchemy was purely for the good of his fellow men. He said that artisans were all alchemists, transmuting the useless into the useful: for example, a baker since he transformed dough into bread; a weaver since he transformed raw cotton, silk and wool into cloth, and so on, according to Pamela Smith in 2004.

Without the alchemists' futile search for the Philosopher's Stone, the cloth industry might never have acquired their compounded dyes. Justus von Liebig said: "In order to know that the Philosopher's Stone did not really exist, it was indispensable that every substance accessible should be observed and examined," according to Ball in 2001. This constant experimentation led to many useful discoveries, such as the transformation of sand and ash to glass through the application of fire. In Renaissance Florence alchemical ideas permeated almost all humanistic pursuits: literature, poetry, fine art and philosophy. Through alchemy scientific research, especially chemistry, evolved.

But the alchemists themselves shrouded their writings in secrecy, using symbolic, magical, ritualistic images that made it difficult to penetrate their secrets.

Cosimo was brilliant at self publicity, channelling his interest in alchemy, which he used to create his herbal medicines, into the creation of a public image of a charitable prince, concerned with the health of his subjects. His courtiers spread the idea that he spent a great deal of time in his *fonderie*, making herbal medicines, but in fact he was involved in so many other projects that he could not have done more than step into them to give instructions to his workers from time to time. However, the idea of a prince making medicines with his own hands and giving them away to courtiers and foreign princes was infinitely appealing. He let everyone know that he studied plants for medicinal use, that he promoted the study of medicine in Pisa University and funded the botanic gardens in Pisa and Florence, all of which added to his prestige, both in Florence and abroad.

Cosimo's Botanical Garden in Florence

Cosimo decided that, since it would be impossible to expand the tiny Santa Maria Nuova Hospital herb garden, he should commission a new large Botanical Garden in Florence. So in 1545 he asked Niccolò Tribolo to design the Garden of San Marco, also known as the *'Giardino delle Stalle'* (the Stables Garden) and Ghini to take charge of planting it, according to Professor F Fabri. Cosimo wanted the students of medicine who were matriculated in Pisa, but returned home to Florence for the long vacations, to continue to study living healing plants on their return. The garden soon had a reputation for rare plants. Tribolo created a quadripartite layout which was used subsequently for many botanical gardens built in the succeeding years.

I decided to go in search of the Florence Botanic Garden in Via Pier Antonio Micheli, right behind the Dominican Friary in Piazza San Marco, where Beato Angelico (Fra Angelico) decorated the walls with his beautiful frescos. It was a sunny day when I stepped into the garden which was surprisingly extensive. It covers 2.3 hectares, with large greenhouses incorporated into monumental buildings, housing lush, tropical plants in rather small terracotta pots. The outside walls of the tropical greenhouse, painted yellow ochre, were speckled white where patches of paint were peeling off, the roof squares of glass were dull grey, in places clouded like cataracts. Funding for the upkeep of the garden does not seem to stretch to cover the maintenance of the buildings.

Turning away from the greenhouse buildings I faced a series of square plots spread out in front of me, some containing plants in pots, some with small fruit trees and some with large mature trees. I came across a green lawn sprinkled with daisies and surrounded by juniper, hawthorn with tiny new leaves, a pomegranate tree just starting to bud, blackthorn in flower and laurel. All except the laurel had been pruned drastically to keep them as small examples.

Gravel paths between the plots were lined with pretty flowering bushes in large terracotta pots. The garden has 4,200 species of plant, most cultivated in terracotta pots in the six small greenhouses, then taken outside in the summer. Not all the plants in the garden today are medicinal but those that are belong to twenty four families. There are fields of bushes, such as elder, chaste tree and myrtle. I came across a border of rosemary bushes covered in clusters of purple flowers, thyme, many different types of sage with spreading silver green foliage, including an enormous Jerusalem sage, all buzzing with bees. *Melissa, Lavandula dentata* and other aromatic plants were bursting into flower and the brilliant blue of *Teucrium frutins* brightened up the border. Other plants were just emerging tentatively from the soil. All the plants had been pruned to round bushes, some mere remnants of last year's growth, some sprouting vigorous new growth.

I came to a field of bulbs, including large quantities of Spanish bluebells, gladiolus, hyacinths and narcissus, interlaced by daisy-like flowers that looked like confetti. There is a field of three hundred different species of mature oak trees, some small and some large and stately. Another field was full of different species of large, mature pine trees. In the middle of the garden there is a small section of raised beds planted with vegetables, such as *cavolo nero*, celery, fennel, cabbage and onion.

It was March, sunny and peaceful, when I went to visit the Florence herb garden, too early in the year to see all the plants, most of which were still lingering in the greenhouses. I could hear birds, distant traffic and occasional nearby traffic and I thought of Cosimo I de' Medici's vision, dedicating some of his banker's money to the creation of this herb garden for the benefit of herbal students but also for the people of Florence, who he felt needed a garden.

Soon after, other European towns and universities created their own botanic gardens.

Cosimo's Garden at Villa di Castello

Cosimo asked Tribolo to restore the garden at his Villa di Castello in 1537. After Tribolo died Vasari took over the layout of the garden. Bernardo Buontalenti took over the restoration work. The garden surrounding the Villa was full of exotic plants and became famous for its elaborate architectural design, the statues, grottoes, fountains and astonishing waterworks. Its scheme was designed for the glorification of the city of Florence and the Medici house. The statues in the garden had to display the greatness and bounty of the house of the Medici and all the Duke's virtues: justice, piety, worth, nobility, knowledge and liberality, according to Vasari in his Vita di Nicolò detto il Tribolo. Cosimo commissioned a statue of Aesculapius: the Greek god of medicine, in the herb garden of the Villa. (For a full description of Aesculapius see my book: *Healing Plants of Greek Myth.*)

Vasari describes a large alley 'covered on its sides and above, in its height of ten "braccia," with a continuous vault of mulberry trees and the labyrinth made of cypresses, laurels, myrtles and box, a garden of orange trees and a *salvatico* of cypresses, firs, ilex and other evergreens.' Claudio Tolomei's letter of 1543, quoted in Lazzaro, The Italian Renaissance Garden, states: 'now it seems a natural artifice, now artificial nature.' The walls that divided the garden into sections, grottoes and trellises were all covered in vegetation. Trees were often used as architectural elements, as different forms of topiary, tall trees as obelisks. The mulberry tree alley and the labyrinth are described by Pierre Belon (1517–1564) who says that some of the plants were extremely rare, such as the Indian figs (Indian Banyan tree), real planes and some rhododendron (actually oleanders), all recently imported.

Vincenzo Ferrini sent a letter to Pier Francesco Riccio, superintendent of some of the Medici villas, referring to 'a large number of herb plants that his Excellency wants to have planted at Castello.' These were for his garden of simples (medicinal herbs) within the Villa a Castello garden.

When Cosimo retired from public life in 1564 he went to live in his Villa a Castello. He had achieved an enormous amount in a short space of time.

Francesco de' Medici

Cosimo's son Francesco (1541–1587) was a great disappointment to the people of Florence, since he was so obsessed with alchemy that he paid no attention to the needs of the city. He did, however, continue to support the faculty of medicine at Pisa University. In 1555, after Ghini left Pisa, Francesco employed Andrea Cesalpino (1519–1603), an expert botanist and eminent physician, as lecturer of simples (medicinal plants) and director of the Pisa botanical garden. Cesalpino took a keen interest in the botanic garden in Pisa, increasing the number of species in it. He was a published author of works on philosophy, medicine, botany, mineralogy, and history. Comparing botany at the time to an unruly army he said:

> I recognise just this to be the condition of things in the botanical world today, where the vastness and intricacy of the disorder appall the mind, give rise to countless and inextricable errors,

and are the source of endless controversies; for if the genus is not known, no description of a plant, however accurately it may have been transmitted, will enable one to identify it with certainty, and such descriptions are apt to mislead; for if the genera are confused all is confusion, necessarily.

So in 1563, in order to create some kind of order out of this chaos, he created his herbaria, collections of dried plant specimens, which he used to record and preserve plants gathered in the wild. It was the only way to have specimens of all the plants together in one place at one time, since the living plants all flowered at different times of the year. The concept of preserving plant specimens in herbaria is now universally accepted as essential. I remember visiting the enormous herbarium at Kew in London years ago, while carrying out research for my doctorate. I saw retired botanists working in quiet seclusion in an atmosphere of deep concentration.

Cesalpino concentrated on the ways in which plants reproduced, and grouped them into genera and families. His first group was trees and shrubs, the second, plants with exposed seeds, the third, plants with seeds contained in 'vases.' The last group comprised plants that did not seem to have seeds. He then set about classifying them and developed a taxonomic system which he went to great lengths to explain in his *De Plantis,* published in 1583. He said in a letter to the bishop Tornabuoni:

Although the number of plants keeps growing almost constantly and such a number cannot be comprehended by the human intellect, by gathering many of them according to their similarity and so reducing them to a small number, we can easily have knowledge of them as is appropriate.

This new method of studying and classifying plants was the beginning of scientific botany, according to Lyn Thorndike in 1923. Cesalpino pointed out that medicine would benefit from plant classification, as those belonging to the same group often have similar properties, something that modern scientists have found to be true. We now know that plants belonging to the same family tend to contain the same classes of compounds, for example, the Solanaceae all contain tropane alkaloids.

However, Cesalpino did not provide schemes or tables to make his system easy to understand, so his contemporaries did not appreciate his *De Plantis*. It was not until 1682 that Ray in *Methodus Nova* drew up a scheme to clarify Cesalpino's classification. Then in 1738 Linnaeus, who considered Cesalpino's work the first example of systematic botany, wrote his famous *Classes Plantarum,* now considered the basis of plant classification. But it was Cesalpino who first thought of classifying plants into genus and family, based on the organs of nutrition and reproduction.

It was thanks to Medici support for the chair of *materia medica* in the university of Pisa that Luca Ghini and Andrea Cesalpino were able to bring about such progress in the world of botany.

Francesco accumulated a great library of books on alchemy and philosophy, absorbed the philosophical ideas of Rupescissa, Ficino and many other alchemical writers and wished to carry out the great work himself. He commissioned Giorgio Vasari to create a *studiolo*: a laboratory in Palazzo Vecchio, for his alchemical experiments, with two paintings to adorn it. The first picture by Johannes Stradanus (1523–1605) was of an alchemical laboratory. While Stradanus was painting the picture, Francesco was already commissioning a new, much larger, alchemical laboratory: the Casino di San Marco.

Georgiana Hedesan explains that Stradanus's picture, supposedly based on Francesco's laboratory in Palazzo Vecchio, shows him working among his artisans, under the watchful guidance of a physician. Stradanus's painting shows the laboratory revolving around the production of the quintessence, with the still for its production at the front of the picture, the physician pointing to it and Francesco looking at it. The angelic central character in the painting, with his blond hair and feminine features, is the embodiment of the gold quintessence, which he holds in his hands. The painting makes clear that the alchemical production of the quintessence is the most important activity in the laboratory and this is portrayed in idealistic terms.

Francesco wanted to produce a universal medicine or supreme panacea, working with Ficino's idea that the Spiritus Mundi quintessence was the spirit of gold, distilled using the spirit of wine (pure alcohol.) At the back of the picture is another, much larger, still, used to produce quasi-industrial quantities of plant distillates.

Stradanus's second painting for the *studiolo* is of Mercury and Ulysses on Circe's island, where she turned his companions into swine. Mercury gives Ulysses the mysterious herb Moly to prevent Circe from transforming him. In Renaissance Florence the word Moly referred to a poison antidote consisting of many different herbs. Mattioli, who was close to the Medici court, produced a famous scorpion oil antidote which probably inspired Cosimo and Francesco to produce their own version. The depiction of Ulysses receiving Moly may obliquely hint at the Medici scorpion oil.

In addition to his Studiolo, Francesco transformed Cosimo I's public offices in the Uffizi building into an art gallery and a collection of art and alchemy laboratories, where artists and scientists worked and collaborated. Clearly this demonstrated how little interest he had in running the city. However, it was of benefit to goldsmiths, jewellers, sculptors, painters and precious stone cutters, who all exchanged equipment and knowledge, both theoretical and technical with the alchemists they were working alongside.

In 1575 Francesco moved most of the equipment and artisans from his studiolo in Palazzo Vecchio to the Casino di San Marco. He spent a great deal of time there, as ambassador Andrea Gussoni remarked:

[Francesco] takes great delight in working with alembics producing many waters and oils apt to treat many diseases and he has a remedy for almost all of them. And among others he makes an oil of such excellent virtue that using it externally on the wrists, heart, stomach, and throat, protects them and cures any sort of poison, heals the plague-stricken, and is a most efficacious remedy for petechiae and any kind of malignant fever; and I was told that he wanted to experiment with it on persons that had been sentenced to death; he made them drink poison and then using this oil he cured them.

There was, in fact, no cure for the plague. Almost everyone infected died. A few people recovered and a few people did not catch it. Anyone who could afford to leave the city when the plague arrived did so. Lorenzo the Magnificent removed his family from Florence when the 1478 plague began. Boccaccio was one of the survivors of the 1348 plague that destroyed a quarter of the people living in Florence. This inspired him to write the Decameron, a story about seven men and three women who escape the disease by fleeing to a villa outside the city. This leads us to question the validity of Gussoni's remarks.

In 1577 Francesco invited Jacopo Ligozzi (1547–1627), the most talented and refined painter of natural things, to Florence and provided him with his own workshop in the Casino di San

Marco, where he painted a large number of plants and animals. Almost all of these are in the *Gabinetto dei Disgni e Delle Stampe* in the Uffizi. Mina Bacci said:

> By comparison with the pictures painted by artists who were paid a salary by Aldrovandi... Ligozzi's paintings reveal at once a much higher quality that distinguishes them immediately even from the best of Aldrovandi's painters.

Ligozzi was just one of the many artists and artisans who worked in the Casino di San Marco, creating ceramics, glassware, jewellery, enamelware, paintings and sculptures.

Francesco asked Buontalenti to help him create a garden at the villa di Pratolino on an unprepossessing site. Together they managed to create a strange and magical garden of vegetation, flowing water, grottoes, fountains, sculptures and automatons. There were tables and seats on the branches of an enormous oak tree and rare plants in a secret garden. Ulisse Aldrovandi admired a fine horse chestnut, *Castanea equina* or (*Aesculus hippocastanum.*) Unfortunately this fabulous garden was abandoned in the nineteenth century.

There were many other private gardens in and around Florence belonging to aristocratic families such as the Salviati, the Bandini, the Scali and the Vecchietti. Cavalier Niccoló Gaddi created a garden of rare and medicinal plants that became known as Gaddi's Paradise. The renowned botanist, Giuseppe Benincasa came to visit Gaddi and through him met Francesco, who invited him to join the Medici court, calling him a herbalist or *Herbarius*. He asked him to find new plants and oversee their acclimatisation in the garden of the Casino di San Marco and later in the Florence Botanic Garden. Benincasa settled in Florence and helped Francesco to expand Cosimo's botanic gardens.

Ferdinando de' Medici

When he was a cardinal Ferdinando (1541–1609) lived in a villa on Pincio Hill in Rome, surrounded by a garden of medicinal plants, dwarf fruit trees and trellises of rare citruses. When Francesco died in 1587 he returned to Florence, became the next Grand Duke of Tuscany and set about restoring the reputation of dynasty, so tarnished by Francesco's neglect. He funded the arts and sciences, including natural history, and created gardens, as Lorenzo and Cosimo I had done before him. One of his first projects was to restore the Villa l'Ambrogiana and its vast quadripartite gardens, between Florence and Pisa. During the sixteenth century new plants continued to arrive from the Americas and from Asia and the Levant, so more and more different species became available. Ferdinando was enthusiastic about the new species and grew them in his gardens.

He put Niccolò Gaddi in charge of the Florence botanical garden and encouraged him to develop it. Later he entrusted the work to Benincasa, sending him on herb collecting expeditions all over Italy and even as far away as Crete. In 1591 Benincasa wrote to Ferdinando:

A most happy chance has befallen me, that is, (I have met) a young German (Georg Dyckmann) with whom I have come to an agreement that during this trip he will paint for me all of the plants from life on royal paper for an honest price including expenses, and he is quite talented in this profession and I trust will make a beautiful work, which will be (complemented) with descriptions of (all these plants), and in this way I hope to do honour to your Most Serene Lordship.

Ferdinando immediately agreed to fund Dyckmann's paintings, thus making it possible for Benincasa to compile a visual record of many species he found on the island. He returned to Florence with his collection of rare plants and botanical illustrations. Ferdinando was delighted with the results of the expedition and sent Benincasa to Pisa to oversee the creation of a new and larger botanical garden, closer to the university than the original one. Benincasa encouraged botanical illustration while he was in charge of the Pisa garden, inviting Daniello Froeschl to come and paint medicinal and rare plants when they were in flower. Froeschl and Benincasa created an artists' studio in the grounds of the Pisa botanical garden. Benincasa died in 1595 but the Medici continued to support the many artists who came to work in the Pisa botanical garden studio, right up until 1630, when yet another episode of the plague destroyed the economy and the garden was abandoned.

After Ferdinand's death his illegitimate son Antonio inherited the Casino and a passion for medical alchemy. He continued to accumulate a library of alchemical recipes.

Part 2

Healing Plants of the Renaissance

In my search for healing plants of Renaissance Florence I discovered a book by Cristina Bellorini: *The World of Plants in Renaissance Tuscany*; that focusses on plants used as medicine in Tuscany in the second half of the sixteenth century. This was the period when the great Cosimo I de' Medici and his sons, Francesco and Ferdinando, were the rulers of Florence and Tuscany. Cristina made a detailed study of the account books of the apothecary shop, the *Speziale al Giglio*, in the archive of the *Ospedale degli Innocenti* in Florence. She focussed on the period when the shop was supplying medicines to the Medici court, especially to Cosimo I. She encountered problems deciphering recipes for mixtures of herbs and had to consult the *Ricettariao Fiorentino*: the *Florentine Pharmacopoeia*, for lists of the ingredients these recipes contained. Sometimes she came across multiple examples of a recipe with the same name but different lists of ingredients.

However, she was able to extract a list of the ingredients most frequently mentioned in 1568, such as sugar and honey, which were used to preserve the medicaments and make them taste better. Cassia and senna were widely used as laxatives, sometimes mixed with other herbs, such as tamarind, rhubarb, violets, aniseed, liquorice. Chicory was often used as a syrup, or a decoction for diluting various other preparations. Chamomile was another popular herb, valued for its calming effect. They used almonds a great deal.

She was struck by the discrepancy between the *Florentine Pharmacopoeia*, which included more than four hundred medicinal plants, and the apothecary shop books which only mentioned a hundred and two. She suggested that the herbs listed in the apothecary shop books were probably the most commonly used herbs. She listed the Italian names of these plants, together with the number of times they appeared in the books for the year 1568. I took her list as a starting point, eliminating all the plants whose names I was unable to translate into English, then selecting twenty five native to Italy and nine exotic plants, most of which could still be used today.

The apothecary occasionally used minerals, such as zinc oxide for ointments, and various animal substances, but on the whole they tended to focus on plants.

Medicinal plants were hardly ever used or sold on their own, though the Grand duke ordered batches of individual plants for his alchemical workshop. The apothecary made up mixtures of plants, either in the form of readymade drugs or for people to process at home, just as herbalists and traditional healers do today. They created syrups, waters, decoctions, pills, juleps, electuaries, suppositories, steam inhalations, oils, unguents, plasters, and herbs to add to baths. Syrups were the most popular, especially rose syrup. The *spezeria* also sold betony and chicory syrups. Waters were divided into natural waters from rain, wells, springs and thermal baths; and waters of distilled herbs, such as rose water, betony water, chicory water, chamomile water and so on. Waters were used to dilute purges. Decoctions were also used to dilute purges. Pills were made from dried, compressed herbs mixed with syrups, waters or decoctions and formed into pills. People sometimes used sponges to apply external remedies.

Chapter 1

Aloe
Aloe vera

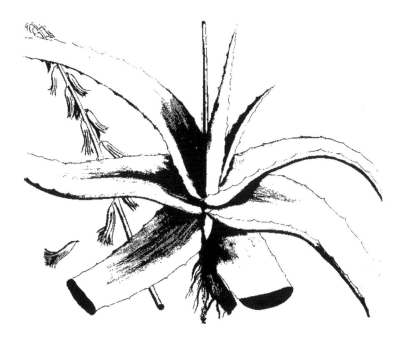

Aloe is mentioned nine times in the Speziale al Giglio: the apothecary shop, but there is no way of knowing which species of Aloe the Florentine physicians were using. I have chosen to focus on *Aloe vera* because I have long been a fan, always keeping a plant growing on my south-facing window sill. I once made the mistake of leaving one outside in the frost. It turned into a drooping sludgy wreck. Away from the frost these plants will grow and thrive for years on end. Whenever anyone in the house burns themselves, whether in the kitchen or outside in the sun, I cut a leaf off, slice it open and smear the gelatinous contents onto the affected part. By the next day the burn is miraculously healed.

Botanical Description

Aloes are succulent plants belonging to the Lilly family with perennial, strong, fibrous roots and numerous leaves, which grow from the upper part of the root. The leaves are narrow, tapering, thick and fleshy with spiny teeth at the edges. Many of the species are woody and branching. Aloes produce flowers in erect, terminal spikes. The flowers are red and have no calyx but a tubular corolla, divided into six segments at the mouth. The true aloe is in flower most of the year and is not to be confused with the Agave, or American Aloe. The inner part of the leaf is a clear, soft, moist, slippery tissue that consist of large, thin-walled cells in which water is held as a viscous mucilage.

Healing Properties

Aloe vera is anti-inflammatory, anti-bacterial, anti-viral, antiseptic, wound healing and protects the skin.

Chemistry

Aloe vera contains polysaccharides which form a water-retaining gel with wound-healing properties. It contains minerals: calcium, chlorine, chromium, copper, iron, magnesium, manganese, potassium, phosphorous, sodium, zinc; amino acids: alanine, arginine, aspartic acid, glutamic acid, glycine, histidine, hydroxyproline, isoleucine, leucine, lysine, methionine, phenylalanine, proline, threonine, tyrosine, valine. It contains phenolic compounds, organic acids, vitamins: B1, B2, B6, beta carotene, choline, folic acid and vitamin E. The bitter yellow substance which can be squeezed out of the leaves contains 1,8 dihydroxy-anthraquinone derivatives and their glycosides, which are purgative. It contains five phytosterols and the purgative aloin.

Research

In 2019 Hekmatpou and Mehrabi reviewed clinical trials which demonstrated that *Aloe vera* healed skin wounds. They found that it had been used to prevent skin ulcers and to treat burn wounds, postoperative wounds, cracked nipples, genital herpes, psoriasis and chronic wounds, including pressure ulcers. They concluded that it can be used to retain skin moisture and will improve wound healing. The healing effect of *Aloe vera* is due to a compound: mannose-6-phosphate, that causes the wound to contract and stimulates collagen synthesis. The polysaccharides in Aloe vera also speed up the healing process. According to the American Botanical Council in 2016 a clinical trial demonstrated that the gel healed wounds earlier than a standard treatment (1% silver sulfadiazine cream). The gel also modulates the immune system. Scientists demonstrated that it reduced inflammation in rats. Scientists have shown that *Aloe vera* gel decreased the size of wounds and speeded up healing.

Fermented Aloe vera gel inhibits pathogenic bacteria, without harming healthy gut bacteria. The compound aloin in it has a laxative effect. The phytosterols in the gel reduce the accumulation of fat in the viscera, and reduce the size of intestinal polyps. The anthraquinone, aloe emodin and the phytosterols in the gel may have an anti-diabetic effect. The gel is also anti-inflammatory and antioxidant, possibly because it contains vitamins E and C, phenolic compounds and polysaccharides. The phytosterols in the gel protect the liver and help it to break down fats. The anthraquinones (aloin and aloe-emodin) have anticancer effects. The physterols in the gel have oestrogenic effect and may be effective at preventing polycystic ovary syndrome.

Scientists have demonstrated that *Aloe vera* gel is anti-bacterial, anti-fungal and anti-viral, probably due to the anthraquinones in it, since they are similar to the antibiotic tetracycline, which inhibits bacteria from reproducing. The polysaccharides in it stimulate immune cells to destroy bacteria. The gel may be effective for treating ulcers. Scientists have demonstrated that the gel improves the immune response of people with HIV since it prevents the virus from entering the cells.

How to Use Aloe

The gel from the inside of the leaves is invaluable for every kind of burn, including sunburn and for speeding up the healing of wounds. I would recommend growing a plant on your windowsill to use whenever anyone burns themselves.

Contraindications

I would not recommend taking *Aloe vera* internally although it contains minerals and vitamins, because there is a potential cancer risk and it may damage the blood, the central nervous system and sperm. *Aloe vera* that has been treated to remove the anthraquinones is safe.

Chapter 2

Aniseed
Pimpinella anisum

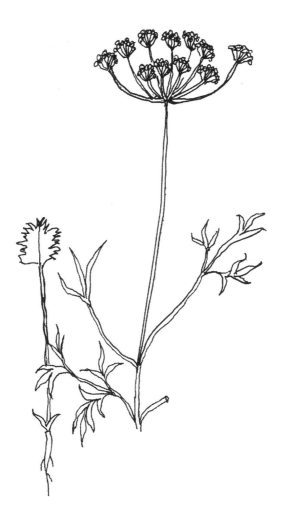

Aniseed appears eight times in the Spezeria al Giglio. Years ago our neighbours from Marseilles used to sit in what once may have been a garden behind the house we were staying in in rural

France. Surrounded by brambles, nettles and high grass, they sat at their little table drinking cloudy glasses of Pastis. Come and join us, they called to me. Come and have a drink of Pastis. I really didn't fancy the strong taste of aniseed, but clearly they loved it. Maybe this was a Marseilles thing, I thought.

Botanical Description

Aniseed is a dainty plant belonging to the Umbelliferae, 60–90 centimetres tall, with a grooved stem. The leaves at the base of the plant are simple, 1–5cm long and shallowly lobed, with a toothed edge and petioles which can be 4–10cm long. The leaves higher on the stems are feathery or lacy, pinnate and divided into numerous small alternately arranged bright green feathery leaflets. Leaves and flowers grow in large, loose clusters. The flowers are either white or yellow, approximately 3 millimetres in diameter, produced in dense umbels. The seed is dry, oblong, curved 4–6mm long and usually called "aniseed"

Healing Properties of Aniseed

Aniseed tea is anti-spasmodic, so will cure abdominal cramps, flatulence and a disturbed digestive system. It is expectorant, so a valuable addition to cough mixtures. According to Rajab in 2016, aniseed is antibacterial and anti-fungal, can reduce inflammation and may reduce feelings of depression. It soothes sore throat, tonsillitis and headache. It may activate the immune system. It also facilitates childbirth and increases milk yield in nursing mothers.

Chemical Constituents

Aniseed contains 1.5–6% volatile oil, consisting mainly of trans-anethole, plus anisaldehyde, estragole, and linalool; 8–11% fatty acids, such as palmitic and oleic acids, 4% carbohydrates and 18% protein, according to Besharati-Seidani in 2005.

Research

In 2002 Singletary reviewed the research that has been carried out into the healing properties of aniseed. He gathered data from a variety of scientific methods such as cell culture experiments and animal studies which demonstrated that aniseed was antioxidant, anti-inflammatory, and antimicrobial. For example, in 2008 Akhtar demonstrated that aniseed was antibacterial *in vitro*. In 2012 Shojaii and Mehri Abdollahi Fard found that aniseed was antibacterial, anti-fungal, insecticidal and anti-viral *in vitro*. The essential oil was anti-spasmodic, anticonvulsant and analgesic. Laboratory experiments showed that it would relax muscles.

A few human clinical trials, mostly in Iran, where aniseed is used in traditional medicine, demonstrate that aniseed might help to allay the signs and symptoms of diabetes, gastro-intestinal distress, sinusitis, migraines, dysmenorrhea, and menopausal hot flashes. For example, in 2008 Nahidi carried out a double blind clinical trial on 72 postmenopausal women. Aniseed extracts seemed to reduce the frequency and intensity of their hot flashes. In 2015 Ashraffodin Ghoshegir and team carried out a double blind clinical trial on 107 people. They found that three grams of anise powder after meals three times a day relieved the symptoms of dyspepsia and even continued to do so eight weeks after the end of the trial. In 2016 Mosaffa-Jahromi and team carried out a double blind randomised clinical trial on 120 patients suffering from irritable bowel syndrome. They divided them into three groups and gave them either: AnisEncap (enteric coated capsules of anise oil), placebo or Colpermin®. They found that the enteric coated capsules of anise oil were a safe treatment for irritable bowel syndrome and more effective than Colpermin®. In 2019 Hamdollah Mosavata Abbas carried out a randomised placebo-controlled trial on fifty patients suffering from migraine. They rubbed a cream, containing essential oil of aniseed, into the skin. They found that it relieved the symptoms of migraine. In 2019 Faramand and team's clinical trial on 67 young women demonstrated that 110mg capsules of Anise three times a day helped to decrease the symptoms of premenstrual syndrome compared with a placebo. These trials were on small numbers of people, so not statistically significant, but they do indicate that aniseed may be a useful healing plant. Further and larger clinical trials should be carried out.

How to Use Aniseed

Make a tea from a teaspoon of the crushed seeds steeped in boiling water for five minutes to cure stomach ache, flatulence and settle disturbed digestion. Herbalists add it to cough mixtures. Use aniseed essential oil diluted in a carrier oil for massage to relieve PMS and headache. You could, of course, drink a small glass of an aniseed liqueur, such as French Pastis, Greek Ouzo or Italian Sambuca mixed with water.

Contraindications

Be careful not to take too much aniseed. Avoid aniseed during pregnancy and breastfeeding. Do not take aniseed if you are taking birth control pills or tamoxifen. Do not take aniseed if you are allergic to asparagus, caraway, celery, coriander, cumin, dill or fennel. Do not ingest aniseed essential oil. 1–5ml aniseed essential oil can cause nausea, vomiting and pulmonary oedema.

Chapter 3

Chamomile
Matricaria chamomilla and *Chamomilla recutita*

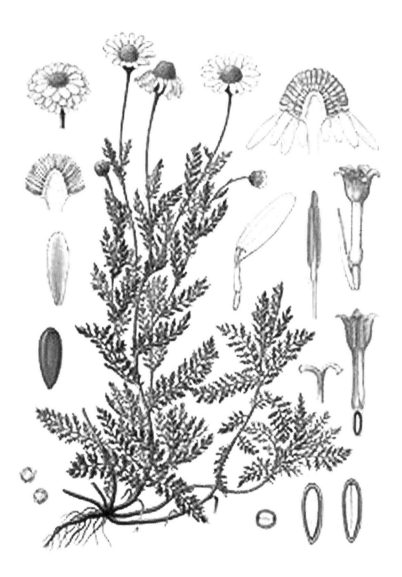

Chamomile is mentioned sixteen times in the Florentine *spezeria* account books. The Florentines may have used the Roman and/ or the German species. I feel sure that Cosimo would have acquired the German as well as the Roman chamomile but, of course, the *spezeria* account books do not specify which they sold since botanical identification did not yet exist. Mattioli said that chamomile was hot and dry and had many medicinal virtues, was calming and soothed the digestion.

Botanical Description

German chamomile, a member of the *Matricaria* genus, is low-growing and branches out, while Roman chamomile, a member of the *Chamaemelum* genus, grows upright on single stems. Roman chamomile is perennial, whereas German chamomile is annual. German chamomile has light green leaves, which tend to have a fern-like appearance. However, Roman chamomile typically has greyish-green leaves, which are thicker and flatter than those of German chamomile. Both German and Roman chamomile have hairy, branching stems covered with leaves which are divided into fine, thread-like segments which give the plants a feathery appearance. Roman chamomile flowers are slightly larger and more substantial than those of German chamomile. The central discs on Roman chamomile are rounded, while on German chamomile, they are hollow yellow cones with white petals drooping down from them. Additionally, the flowers on German chamomile grow as a single flower on each stem, while on Roman chamomile, they branch out and grow as several flowers on each stem.

Healing Properties

Chamomile is carminative, sedative and tonic. An infusion of the dried flowers makes an excellent remedy for children suffering from earache, neuralgic pain, stomach ache, or just general nervousness, since it is gentle and non-toxic yet has a wonderful calming effect. People use chamomile for hay fever, inflammation, muscle spasms, menstrual disorders, insomnia, ulcers, wounds, gastrointestinal disorders, rheumatic pain, and haemorrhoids. The German Commission E recommends chamomile infusion.

Chemical Constituents

Chamomile contains 0.24–1.9% volatile oil, which ranges in colour from brilliant blue to deep green when fresh but turns dark yellow after it has been stored. It does not lose its potency. The main compounds in the essential oil are alpha-bisabolol terpenoids and oxide azulenes, including chamazulene, which is unstable and best preserved in alcoholic tincture. It also contains lactones, glycosides, hydorxycoumarins and flavonoids: apigenin, luteolin, patuletin an quercetin. It contains coumarins: herniarin and umbelliferone; terpenoids and mucilage.

Research

In 1994 Merfort demonstrated that chamomile flavonoids and essential oils penetrated the skin of human volunteers, which is important since people use chamomile essential oil diluted in a carrier as a massage for inflammatory pain or congestive neuralgia.

Several scientists have investigated the anti-cancer activity of the chamomile compound, apigenin, including Way, in 2004, who found that it destroyed breast cancer cells, Birt in 1997, who demonstrated that it inhibited the growth of skin cancer cells and Gates in 2007, who found that people who ate a diet containing large amounts of flavonoids tended not to suffer from ovarian cancer. In 2007 Srivastava demonstrated that chamomile extracts destroyed various types of cancer cells, without affecting normal cells. In 2009 Evans demonstrated that a novel agent, TBS-101, a mixture of seven herbal extracts, including chamomile, inhibited prostate cancer in animal models.

Common cold is the most common human disease. People have known for centuries that filling a bowl with boiling water, dropping a few chamomile flowers onto the surface, then inhaling the steam, would relieve the symptoms of nasal congestion. In 1990 Saller demonstrated that inhaling steam with chamomile extract helped to relieve common cold symptoms.

Several scientists, including Hertog in 1993, suggest that people who eat a lot of food containing flavonoids (fruit and vegetables) are less likely to suffer from coronary heart disease. In 1973 Gould demonstrated that blood flow to the brachial arteries increased in patients who drank chamomile tea before cardiac catheterisation. Ten of the twelve patients fell into a deep sleep soon after drinking the tea.

In 2007 Gardiner gave a herbal tea containing chamomile, vervain, liquorice, fennel, balm and mint to thirty four infants suffering from colic and a placebo to another thirty-four infants. After seven days parents reported that the herbal tea eliminated the colic in 57% of the infants, whereas the placebo was helpful in 26%. In 1997 Kell gave chamomile extract and apple pectin to thirty-nine infants and placebo to another forty suffering from diarrhoea and found that the diarrhoea ended more quickly in the infants receiving the chamomile and pectin.

In 1988 Nissen found that chamomile cream was moderately effective against eczema. In 1983 Albring demonstrated that it was about 60% as effective as hydrocortisone cream. The Manzana type of Roman chamomile is rich in active ingredients but does not cause allergies in the same way as the German chamomile does. In 2000 Petzelt-Wenczler demonstrated that a cream containing Manzana chamomile (Kamillosan(R) cream) was more effective than hydrocortisone cream. Further research is needed to see whether chamomile could be used to manage eczema.

People use chamomile to treat upset stomach, spasm, colic, flatulence, ulcers and gastrointestinal irritation, according to Kroll in 2006. It's especially helpful for dispelling gas, soothing the stomach, and relaxing the muscles that move food through the intestines. In 2006 Khayyal demonstrated that a commercial preparation (STW5, Iberogast), containing the extracts of bitter candy tuft, lemon balm leaf, chamomile flower, caraway fruit, peppermint leaf, liquorice root, angelica root, milk thistle fruit and greater celandine herb, was an effective treatment for ulcers and rebound acidity. It reduced the acid in the intestine and increased the secretion of mucilage, which protects the walls of the intestines.

In 2003 Lyseng-Williamson suggested that chamomile ointment might improve haemorrhoids. Adding tincture of chamomile to a sitz bath may also reduce haemorrhoid inflammation.

In 2005 Wang gave five cups of chamomile tea to fourteen volunteers for two weeks. He found that the volunteers had increased levels of hippurate and glycine in their urine, which indicated that their bodies were fighting bacteria more effectively. They suggested that drinking chamomile tea boosted the immune system.

People have been drinking chamomile tea and using chamomile essential oil aromatherapy to treat insomnia for centuries. In 2005 Shinomiya demonstrated that chamomile and passiflora extracts had a calming effect on rats. In 1999 Paladini demonstrated that inhaling flavonoids, including apigenin, reduced the stress-hormone, ACTH, in the same way as diazepam. Giving diazepam together with apigenin increased the sedative effect. Chamomile contains other compounds in addition to apigenin which may also have a sedative effect. In 2009 Amsterdam carried out a clinical trial which demonstrated that chamomile extract had a modest anti-anxiety effect.

In 2008 Kato demonstrated that chamomile suppressed blood sugar levels and increased glycogen storage in human blood cells. He suggested that it might help allay the side effects of diabetes. In 2008 Cemek demonstrated that chamomile protected the pancreas of diabetic rats.

In 1987 Glowania carried out a clinical trial with 14 patients who had their tattoos scraped off. They found that chamomile speeded up the wound healing. In 2007 Nayak demonstrated that *Matricaria recutita* chamomile extract speeded up wound healing. In 2009 Martins demonstrated in vitro and in vivo that *Chamomilla recutita* healed wounds faster than corticosteroids.

How to Use Chamomile

Chamomile is a gentle, soothing herb. Make a tea with a teaspoonful of dried chamomile flowers and give to infants with colic, possibly sweetened with honey. For a stronger effect make an infusion with 30g of dried flowers, steeped in a pint of boiled water for five minutes. Cover to prevent the healing elements from evaporating while it steeps. Drink for its calming effect, especially just before going to bed for a relaxing sleep. Make a massage oil by diluting chamomile essential oil in a carrier oil, such as sunflower and massage to relieve muscle aches, menstrual cramps, inflammation and stomach ache. You could make an ointment by adding chamomile essential oil to an ointment base or you could add a few drops of chamomile essential oil to an ointment made from other healing plants, such as calendula, St John's wort, rose etc. Add a few chamomile flowers to boiled water and inhale to relieve a congested nose when you have a cold. Use a chamomile cream for eczema.

Contraindications

A few people are allergic to chamomile. People who are allergic to chrysanthemums or other members of the composite family tend to be allergic to chamomile, especially if they take other drugs that help to trigger the sensitisation. Do not wash your eyes with chamomile tea if you have hay fever and conjunctivitis. It will make it worse.

Chapter 4

Carob Tree
Ceratonia siliqua

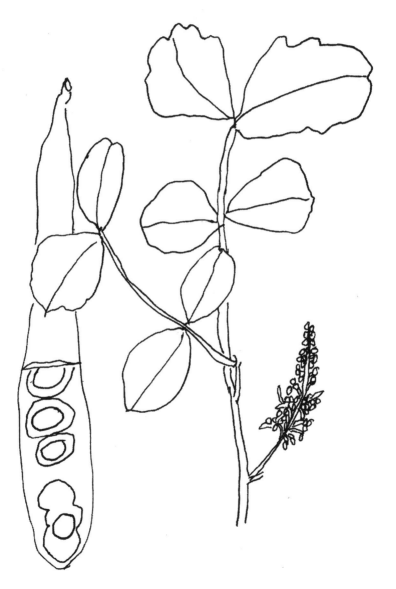

The scientific name of the carob tree (*Ceratonia siliqua* L.) derives from Greek *keras*, horn, and Latin *siliqua*, alluding to the hardness and shape of the pod. The genus *Ceratonia* belongs to the family Leguminosae (or Fabaceae), the bean family, which fixes nitrogen in the soil. The carob tree originated in the Middle-East where the ancient Greeks recognised its value and brought it to Greece and Italy. The Arabs disseminated it along the north African coast and north into Spain and Portugal. It is also called the locust bean tree or St John's bread because it has edible bean pods which people believed were the 'locusts' that St John the Baptist fed on when he was in the desert. People pick the ripe pods, roast and grind them to make carob powder, ferment them to make alcohol, or dilute the powder to make carob syrup. The seeds contain a gum which is used as a food thickener and stabiliser. Farmers sometimes feed the ground pods to their farm animals.

Carob powder is sometimes used as a substitute for chocolate since it has fewer calories and doesn't contain caffeine or theobromine, but it can never be a substitute for dark chocolate. Cacao arrived in Europe during the Renaissance but was an expensive luxury, so carob powder was highly valued.

Botanical Description

The carob tree grows to about fifteen metres with a broad hemispherical crown, a thick trunk and sturdy branches. It has feather-formed, glossy, evergreen, alternate, pinnate leaves 10–20cm long, with or without terminal leaflets. The dark green leaflets have a very thick epidermis containing large amounts of tannins. The small and numerous red flowers grow in clusters directly along the branches. The fruit is a straight or curved pod, 10–30cm long, 1.5–3.5cm broad and 6–20mm thick. The pods have a wrinkled surface that turns dark brown and leathery when they are mature. They contain 5–18 hard brown seeds (10% of the pod weight) embedded in a sweet thick pulpy substance.

Healing Properties

Carob has a calming effect on the digestion and will relieve diarrhoea and heartburn. People use it for absorption disorders such as celiac disease and sprue. It is also used to treat obesity, vomiting during pregnancy, and high cholesterol. People give carob syrup to infants to cure them of vomiting, retching cough, and diarrhoea. Carob might cause weight loss, reduce blood sugar and insulin levels, and lower cholesterol levels. It is anti-oxidant and anti-inflammatory. Based on Agrawal's personal experience he states that molasses of Carob is very active against mouth inflammations.

Chemical Constituents

Carob seed pods contain 90% pulp and 10% seeds. The pulp contains 48–56% total sugars which include sucrose 32–38%, glucose 5–6%, fructose 5–7%, pinitol 5–7%, and small quantities of maltose, raffinose, stachyose, verbascose, and xylose, plus condensed tannins 18–20%, non-starch polysaccharides, fat 2–3% and small amounts of numerous minerals: copper, calcium, manganese, potassium, magnesium, zinc, selenium and vitamins: A, B2, B3, B6. The pods also contain fibre 40%, which includes cellulose, hemicellulose and lignin.

The seed coats contain antioxidants and the endosperm (the inside part of the seed) contains glactomannan, a type of gum composed of polysaccharides. This natural polysaccharide forms a viscous stable solution when highly diluted in water. When the gum is used as a food additive it is known as E 410.

Research

In 2008 Berrougui found that aqueous extracts of carob fruits inhibited inflammation and the oxidation of fats. In

2011 Agrawal demonstrated that extract of carob pods was antidepressant in rats. Mokhtari in 2011 demonstrated the anti-diabetic effect of carob seeds extract. Condensed tannins (CT) can modify carbohydrate digestion and absorption. Since the high concentration of CT in the pulp of carob fruit suggests a potential anti-diabetic effect, several scientists, including Macho-Gonzales in 2017 demonstrated that it decreased diabetic rats' absorption of carbohydrates.

Several scientists have demonstrated the anti-cancer effect of carob pods in the laboratory. In 2017 Amessis-Ouchemoukh found that extracts of *Ceratonia siliqua* pods were antioxidant and anti-cancer. In 2002 Corsi demonstrated that carob pod extracts killed mouse liver cancer cells *in vitro*. Several scientists including Kumazawa in 2002 have demonstrated that aqueous extract of carob pods was antioxidant in the laboratory.

In 2011 Agrawal listed experiments that demonstrated that carob pods protected the digestive system of rats from ulcers and ulcerative colitis. Carob pod extracts also protected rats' livers and diabetic rats' kidneys.

In 1989 Forestieri demonstrated that carob fruit extract lowered blood glucose in rats. In 2020 Macho-Gonzales demonstrated that including carob extract in the diet of diabetic rats improved their insulin resistance. The rats had lower blood glucose levels and higher levels of insulin as well as healthier pancreatic beta cells and better storage of glycogen in the liver. In 2019 Macho-Gonzalez found that carob extract improved levels of fats in the blood of diabetic rats fed on a high fat diet. He also found that their blood sugar levels fell and insulin levels rose.

There have been a few clinical trials demonstrating that eating carob-based foods helps people to feel less hungry. In 2017 Papakonstantinou carried out a single-blinded, randomised, crossover trial, giving 40g of carob snack to half the participants and 40g of chocolate cookie to the other half. Fifty healthy, non-diabetic normal-weight men took part. Results showed that the men who ate the carob snack consumed significantly less carbohydrate during the subsequent twenty four hours, felt fuller and less hungry and were less preoccupied with thoughts of food than those who ate the chocolate cookie.

Carob seems to lower fats in the bloodstream. In 2020 Jaffari divided forty obese men into four groups: resistance training, 1.5g carob supplement per day, combined resistance training and carob supplement and control group. The group who did the resistance training together with the carob supplement had a significantly improved level of fats in their blood. In 2003 Zunft carried out a randomised, double-blind placebo-controlled trial with fifty eight adults suffering from high levels of cholesterol. He gave half the participants 15g of carob for six weeks. He found that total cholesterol, triglycerides and low density lipoprotein (bad fats) decreased in those who took the carob. In 2010 Ruiz-Roso demonstrated in his randomised, double-blind, placebo-controlled trial of 97 patients with high cholesterol that eating 8g of carob pulp, rich in fibre, for four weeks, resulted in lowering total cholesterol, triglycerides and low density lipoproteins in the blood of those who ate the carob.

Unfortunately most of the reviewed trials used insufficient patient numbers, leading to a low power of analysis. Also very few of these studies included lifestyle factors such as diet and exercise that could affect the study outcome. Large-scale and well-designed randomised placebo-controlled trials are needed to confirm that carob could improve the health of obese people.

How to Use Carob Tree

The U.S. Food and Drug Administration (FDA) approved carob for use in food, pharmaceuticals, and cosmetics.

Carob is available as powder, chips, syrup, extract and dietary pills. Add carob powder to your breakfast cereal to help you feel less hungry during the day, to lower your cholesterol and, provided that you take plenty of exercise and eat a sensible diet, to lose weight. Use carob powder in your cooking instead of chocolate.

Contraindications

There is not enough information about the safety of taking carob if you are pregnant or breast feeding, so avoid consuming greater than food amounts. Carob contains tannins, which decrease the effectiveness of enzymes that help with digestion so be careful not to eat excessive amounts of it.

Chapter 5

Coriander
Coriandrum sativum

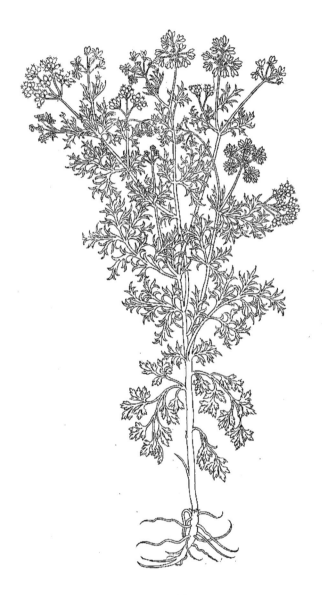

Coriander has a long history, dating back to the Neolithic Age, around 7000 BCE. It is mentioned in Sanskrit texts and the Old Testament and Egyptian papyrus scrolls. The Greeks cultivated it since the second millennium BCE.

My mother used to plant coriander outside the kitchen. It always went to seed and spread everywhere, growing in the cracks in the pathways and all sorts of other places.

In both Chinese and Ayurvedic medicine traditional healers use the seeds to cure digestive complaints and flatulence. Ayurvedic practitioners combine the seeds with caraway and cardamom. European herbalists combine it with caraway, fennel or aniseed to treat digestive complaints such as indigestion, vomiting, diarrhoea, gastrointestinal spasms, dyspepsia, and as an appetite stimulant.

Botanical Description

Coriander is a bright green annual plant between 30–90cm high with many branches growing out of the stem. The lowest leaves have stalks with many roundish leaflets, slightly lobed. The uppermost leaves are linear and more divided. The flowers are asymmetrical, with the petals pointing away from the centre. They have short stalks and grow in pretty umbels of five to ten rays, pale mauve or white. The seed is almost ovate with two parts and multiple ridges along the surfaces.

Healing Properties

Various parts of the plant, such as seeds, leaves and flowers, contain compounds which are diuretic, anti-convulsant, anti-diabetic, sedative, anti-mutagenic, anti-fungal and anti-bacterial. Coriander seeds and leaves may help lower LDL fats (bad fats,) are full of antioxidants, in the form of vitamins, minerals, carotenoids and polyphenols, which remove free radicals from our bodies, thus helping to prevent cancer. Coriander seeds cure intestinal parasites, soothe upset stomachs, calm the nerves and relieve intestinal gas. They may reduce blood glucose, thus helping to control type two diabetes.

Chemical Constituents

The leaves contain beneficial flavonoids, polyphenols, phenolic acids, proteins, vitamins A, C, K; and minerals: calcium, phosphorus, and iron; fibre and carbohydrates. The seeds contain many phenolic compounds, mainly flavonoids, coumarins and phenol carboxylic acids. Coriander seed oil (0.03-2.6%) contains 60–70% linalool, a terpenoid that is a powerful cellular antioxidant as well as the source of coriander's pleasant smell. It also contains fatty acids, mainly petroselinic acid; limonene, alpha-pinene, gamma-terpinene, p-cymene, citronellol, borneol, camphor, coriandrin, geraniol, dihydro-coriandrin, coriandrons A-E according to Nadeem in 2013. It is a rich source of phytosterols, especially beta-sitosterol, which are antioxidant and help to prevent the uptake of cholesterol.

Research

It's safe to use essential oil of coriander seeds well-diluted in carrier oil to treat superficial skin infections and oozing dermatitis caused by Streptococci. In 2015 Mandal and Mandal reviewed the anti-bacterial, anti-fungal and anti-oxidant properties of coriander. They found that many scientists had proven *in vitro* that both the seeds and leaves were anti-bacterial against many different species of bacteria and were anti-fungal. In 2012 Abascal demonstrated in the laboratory that coriander seed oil inhibited several bacteria, including *Staphylococcus aureus, S haemolytic, Pseudomonas aeruginosa, E coli* and *Listeria monocytogenes*. Coriander leaf oil contains aldehydes which destroy *Candida spp, S aureus, Salmonella typhe, S choleraesuis* and other bacteria.

Both the seeds and the leaves have anti-oxidant activity. In 2011 Aissaoui found that coriander seeds lowered cholesterol in rats. In 2008 Dhanapakiam demonstrated that as well as lowering LDL cholesterol in rats, it increased HDL cholesterol (good cholesterol.)

In 2009 Nakamura demonstrated that linalol, the most abundant terpenoid in coriander seed oil, repressed stress in rats when they inhaled it. Coriander seed extract is mildly sedative and good for treating mild anxiety and insomnia. In 2012 Momin demonstrated that it made mice sleep for longer. In another study Emamghoreishi found that seed extract decreased anxiety and relaxed the muscles of mice. He suggested that this was due to the quercetin and isoquercetin in the extract. While the results of these animal studies are promising the calming properties of coriander seed have not yet been clinically tested in humans. Coriander leaves have been shown to decrease symptoms of people with arthritis. Rajeshwari In 2012 suggested that this was due to the antioxidant effect of vitamins A and C, phenolic acids and polyphenols in the leaves. In 2011 Pandey showed that extract of the leaves protected rats' livers from damage.

In 2011 Eidi and Eidi found that coriander seed extract increased active beta cells *in vivo*. Beta cells produce insulin, which stimulates cells to take up glucose from the blood. So they suggested that coriander might help control type two diabetes. However, large doses of coriander seeds could cause allergic reactions because they contain furano-coumarins.

Almost all the research on coriander was carried out in the laboratory. In 2015 Mansour and team carried out a triple-blind, placebo-controlled clinical trial on 66 patients suffering from migraine. They found that common medicine plus coriander seed reduced the severity and length of migraine better than common medicine with placebo.

How to Use Coriander

Coriander is easy to grow and happily spreads, so grow your own if you can, to have a fresh supply. In the US the leaves are called cilantro. Add the leaves to salads. Grind the seeds and add them to curries and other cooked foods.

Boil a teaspoon of coriander seeds in two cups of water until the liquid reduces to half, strain and drink the tea for instant relief from bloating, nausea, indigestion and heavy menstrual flow.

Use the essential oil, well diluted in a carrier oil for an anti-stress massage, to calm anxiety and promote deep sleep.

Contraindications

Some people are allergic to coriander.

People with low blood pressure or diabetes should not take large doses of coriander.

Coriander may interfere with medications for high blood pressure, diabetes, drugs that increase photosensitivity or sedative medications.

Chapter 6

Dill
Anethum graveolens

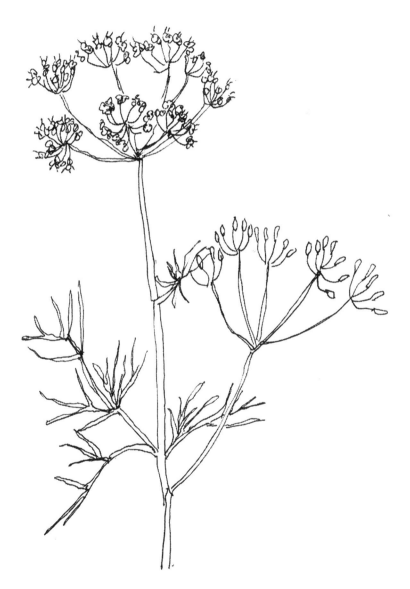

Botanical Description

Dill grows two to two and a half feet high with feathery leaves on sheathing foot stalks with pointed leaflets. It has a long, spindle-shaped root and grows straight up with a smooth, shiny, hollow stem. In midsummer it produces flat umbels of yellow flowers with small petals that roll inwards. It produces great quantities of pungent, bitter seeds. The whole plant is aromatic.

Healing Properties

Dill is used to treat digestive, liver and gallbladder problems, loss of appetite, intestinal gas, bad breath and to reduce cholesterol and blood glucose. It is antimicrobial, anti-inflammatory, anti-oxidant and may help to prevent cancer. The seed is aromatic, carminative, mildly diuretic and stimulates the production of milk.

Chemical Constituents

Dill seeds contain about 36% carbohydrates, 15.68% proteins, 14.80% fibre, 8.39% moisture and 3.5% essential oil: which contains: d-carvone (23.1%) d-limonene (45%). α-phellandrene, eugenol and anethole; fatty oil, minerals, and vitamins; flavonoids: quercetin and isoharmentin; coumarins, triterpenes, phenolic acids and umbelliferones.

The leaves and seeds contain vitamins C, A, folate, riboflavin; minerals: iron, manganese, calcium, copper, magnesium, potassium and zinc.

Research

Most of the research into the healing properties of dill have been carried out in Iran, where traditional healers use it to treat a number of conditions.

Ninety percent of diabetes cases are type two and it is the third most life-threatening disorder in the world. Diabetes results in high blood glucose which causes damage to circulating fats and injury to the blood vessels. It also leads to low levels of high density lipoprotein (HDL) (good fats) and high levels of triglycerides. This doubles, or even quadruples, the risk of heart and cardiovascular disease. In 2016 Goodarzi reviewed the research on how dill is used to control type two diabetes. He found that various scientists had tested dill seed and leaf in the laboratory as a treatment for type two diabetes with promising results. In 2010 Jana significantly reduced triglycerides, cholesterol, low-density lipoprotein (bad fats) and glucose in laboratory experiments. In 2007 Yazdanparast and Bahramikia found that crude extracts of dill lowered cholesterol in rats and reduced the peroxidation of fats in the liver. When free radicals attack fats this causes peroxidation: i.e. damaged fats and inflammation, which causes damage to the blood vessels. They found that dill prevented blood vessel damage *in vivo* and suggested that it might protect the blood vessels of people suffering from high cholesterol. It seems that dill stops cholesterol from being absorbed into the blood. Yazdanparast suggested that carvone, limonene or alpha-phellandrene may be responsible for lowering blood fats. Other studies have suggested that compounds in dill might cause LDL (bad fats) receptors in the liver to increase, thus enabling the liver to absorb and get rid of it. Rutin and quercetin are compounds in dill which may decrease LDL cholesterol. In 2012 Babri suggested that flavonoids, terpenoids, alkaloids tannins and phytosterols in dill may be responsible for lowering cholesterol. The flavonoids and phenolic pro-anthocyanidins are antioxidant.

In 2007 Naseri Gharib and Heidari found that dill seed relaxed the contractions of the intestine *in vivo*, so they suggested that this supported its traditional use for stomach and intestinal disorders.

In 2021 Jalili and team reviewed data from five clinical trials conducted on 227 participants who were given dill: *Anethum graveolens*, for controlling cardiovascular risk and type two diabetes. They found that dill reduced LDL cholesterol, improved cardiovascular health and the patients had less insulin in their blood. In 2020, Haidari and team gave 3g/day dill powder or placebo to forty two patients with type two diabetes. They also found that the patients who took the dill powder had less insulin and LDL cholesterol in their blood, compared with the control group.

In 2014 Heidarifar and team carried out a clinical trial on seventy five young women suffering from severe period pain. They divided the women into three groups and gave one group 500mg of dill seed powder twice a day, one group 250mg mefenamic acid and one group a placebo. They found that the dill seed powder was as effective as the mefenamic acid in reducing the severe pain.

How to Use Dill

Add a tablespoon of dill seeds to a cup of just boiled water. Steep until warm, then drink to calm and sooth your digestion, to get rid of flatulence and acid reflux. To make gripe water to sooth a colicky baby, bruise a tablespoon of dill seeds, boil a cup of water, add the bruised seeds and cover. Allow to cool, then strain out the dill seeds. You could add a little honey. Give the baby a teaspoonful of the gripe water to help them burp. 2–3g of ground dill seeds mixed with water will get rid of worms in children. Drink dill seed tea for a few days before your period is due to relieve menstrual pain and cramping.

Of course you can cook with dill. Add the leafy fronds to egg dishes, cucumber salads, smoked salmon and pickled herrings.

Contraindications

Do not use dill seed as a medicine if you are pregnant or breast feeding. Do not use dill if you are allergic to caraway, celery, coriander or fennel, since you are likely to be allergic to it. Dill seed powder may lower blood sugar, so if you are already taking insulin to control diabetes be very careful to watch for signs of low blood sugar if you take dill. Do not take dill for at least two weeks before undergoing surgery.

Chapter 7

Fennel
Foeniculum vulgare

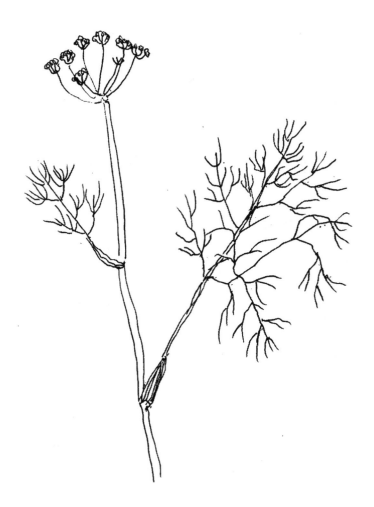

Botanical Description

Fennel is both a vegetable with a bulb-like appearance and a
herb with foliage resembling dill. It is a member of the Apiaceae
family (which also includes carrot) and is grown for its edible

shoots, leaves and seeds. When grown as a herb it has stiff, erect, hollow, branching stems and soft, feathery, almost hair-like foliage growing up to 2m tall. Its stem is bright green, and so smooth that it looks polished, with multiple branched leaves which grow up to 40cm long. They are finely dissected, with threadlike ultimate segments, about 0.5mm wide. The bright golden flowers, produced in large, flat terminal umbels, with thirteen to twenty rays, bloom in July and August. Seeds are oblong to ovoid, 3–5mm long and 1.5–2.0mm broad, elongated with strong ribs. The best fennel seeds are greenish-yellow, the colour of hay, from which the term fennel is derived, with a strong aniseed smell and flavour. Wild fruits are short, dark coloured and blunt at the ends and don't smell or taste as pleasant as the sweet fennel. People use the leaves to dye textiles light green and a combination of leaves and flowers for a brown dye.

Healing Properties

Fennel is anti-bacterial, anti-fungal, anti-viral, anti-parasitic and anti-oxidant so it can be used to bathe cuts, mouth ulcer and conjunctivitis. Compounds in the seeds stimulate the cilia (tiny hairs) in the bronchi to move like brushes, pushing mucous, bacteria, and other matter upwards so that it can be coughed up and spat out. People use the stem, fruit, leaves, seeds, and whole plant medicinally in different forms, including teas, to treat a variety of conditions, including coughs and colds. Fennel essential oil regulates the motility of the smooth muscle of the intestines and reduces gas, so it is good for flatulence, gastritis, dyspepsia, stomachache, abdominal pains, irritable colon, colic in children, nausea, and colitis. People also use it traditionally for arthritis, constipation, fever, insomnia, kidney ailments and liver pain. Animal studies suggest that fennel may protect the liver, lower blood sugar, enhance memory and reduce stress. In Italy they make an aperitif from it, called Finocchietto. The hormone-like compounds in fennel seed may have a beneficial effect on PMS and menopausal symptoms.

Chemical Constituents

Fennel seeds are one of the highest plant sources of potassium, sodium, phosphorus and calcium. They also contain iron, magnesium, zinc and vitamins C, B1, 2, 3 and 6, folate, and vitamins A, E and K. According to USDA data for the Mission variety, fennels are the richest sources of dietary fibre and vitamins. The seeds contain many different polyunsaturated fatty acids and amino acids. Fennel contains essential oil in every part of the plant, which is responsible for its characteristic smell. According to Akgul in 1988, the essential oil contains 87 volatile compounds, mainly trans-anethole, with lesser amounts of estragole and limonene. Fennel, like all members of the Apiaceae family, contains significant quantities of flavonoids, such as quercetin, kaempferol and rosmarinic acid, which are antioxidant and anti-inflammatory, according to Nassar in 2010.

Research

Most of the research into the healing properties of fennel was carried out in laboratories, by scientists all over the world. Several scientists, including Duško, found that extracts of the whole fennel plant and the seeds inhibited many species of bacteria. Many scientists, including Martins in 2012 have demonstrated that fennel is anti-fungal. Several scientists, including Orhan in 2012, have demonstrated that fennel is anti-viral. These results suggest that there is a good reason for people to use fennel to treat infectious conditions such as conjunctivitis, gastritis, mouth ulcer, colds and coughs.

In 2004 Choi demonstrated the anti-inflammatory, analgesic, antioxidant and anti-allergic properties of fennel *in vivo*. In 2003 Ozbek found that fennel essential oil protected the livers of rats.

In 2012 Naga Kishore found that fennel extract had anti-anxiety effect on rats. In 2013 Koppula demonstrated that fennel had an anti-stress effect on rats. It also improved their memory. In 1980 Albert-Puleo found that fennel had an oestrogenic effect in animal studies. He concluded that anethol was responsible. In 2001 Ostad found that fennel essential oil had a strong oestrogen-like effect *in vivo*.

Mohaddese mentions four clinical trials in women with PMS symptoms. In 2007 Nazarpour compared fennel oil with mefenamic acid or placebo. Patients received 20–30 drops of fennel oil every 4–8 hours or mefenamic acid when they started to feel pain during two menstrual cycles. The women did not feel any difference after one cycle, but symptoms improved during second menstrual cycle compared to placebo. In 2011 Delaram carried out a small study on 60 students, comparing fennel oil with placebo in three divided doses three days before and after menstruation for two period cycles. The fennel oil significantly reduced the severity of anxiety, depression and other PMS symptoms, compared to the placebo group. In 2015 Omidali carried out a small trial on 40 women with PMS symptoms, dividing them into four groups and giving them either fennel plus Pilates three times a week, Pilates three times a week, fennel or control for four weeks. They gave the fennel group 30 drops of fennel oil every twelve hours for a month. The group who received fennel oil plus Pilates improved significantly but those who only received fennel didn't. In 2016 Pazoki compared fennel oil, exercise, fennel oil plus exercise and control on 48 students with PMS symptoms. They gave 30 drops of fennel oil every eight hours, three days before and after menstrual cycle. Both the fennel oil and the exercise improved symptoms but the combination of fennel oil and exercise had the best effect. Oestrogens are effective hormones for reducing anxiety and this was proven in 2001 by Pourabbas who gave fennel oil to rats. Mohaddese suggests that fennel oil reduces PMS symptoms because it contains oestrogen-like compounds and because it reduces pain.

Menorrhagia is abnormally heavy or prolonged bleeding during menstruation. In 2003 Khorshidi gave 0.3–1ml fennel oil to patients with dysmenorrhea and it caused the bleeding to increase. On the other hand in 2013 Bokaie found that one hundred drops of fennel oil did not increase bleeding. Eating an 180ml fennel soft capsule daily for two and three months reduced the length of the bleeding.

In 2018 Ghazanfarpour gave fennel oil or sunflower oil twice daily to menopausal women for eight weeks. He noticed that the women who took the fennel oil had less severe night sweating, hot flashes, insomnia and musculo-skeletal disorders after eight weeks compared with placebo group. In 2017 Kian noticed a significant improvement in the symptoms of menopausal women who took a daily dose of 60mg of fennel oil, compared to those on a placebo. In 2018 Ghazanfarpour also found a significant reduction in anxiety in twenty-four post-menopausal women who took 30mg of fennel oil for four weeks compared with control.

A condition that can occur after menopause is atrophic vaginitis: drying and inflammation of the interior of the vagina due to lack of oestrogen. In 2016 Yaralizadeh observed that women suffering from atrophic vaginitis who used a fennel vaginal cream noticed a slight improvement in itching, dryness and pain compared with control. No one carried out a clinical trial using fennel oil topically on atrophic vaginitis. It would be a good idea to investigate this.

Another thing that can happen to women after menopause is male pattern hair growth. In 2014 Akha noticed that women with male pattern hair growth who used creams containing 1% and 2% fennel extract had significantly reduced hair growth, compared to controls. The cream containing 2% was better than the one containing 1%. The oestrogen-like compounds in fennel inhibit the dermal papillae from synthesising dihydrotestosterone. It would be a good idea to investigate how effective creams containing fennel oil are for managing male pattern hair growth.

In 2008 Kim Sang-Moo found that the plaque on the teeth of people treated with the boiled water extract of *F vulgare* decreased significantly compared with controls. They had screened 420 plant extracts for glucosyltransferase (GTase) inhibitors that prevent dental caries. They found that fennel had the highest activity. They suggested that boiled water extracts of fennel could effectively suppress plaque formation.

How to Use Fennel

What little research has been carried out suggests that fennel could be used to allay the symptoms of PMS, menopause, dental caries and numerous other conditions. But the research is incomplete and although eating the vegetable raw or cooked is a thoroughly good idea, I cannot advise anyone to use the essential oil because it has not been proven safe. You can, however, make a tea from fennel seeds to cure stomach ache, especially when caused by flatulence.

Dosage

Fennel seeds 5–7g/day.

Fennel extract vaginal cream (5%) 200mg/day.

Contraindications

Do not take fennel seed oil. Overdosing on it can cause hallucinations and seizures.

Fennel may inhibit cytochrome P450 3A4 so should be used cautiously with medications requiring this isoenzyme as a substrate.

Chapter 8

Fumitory
Fumaria officinalis

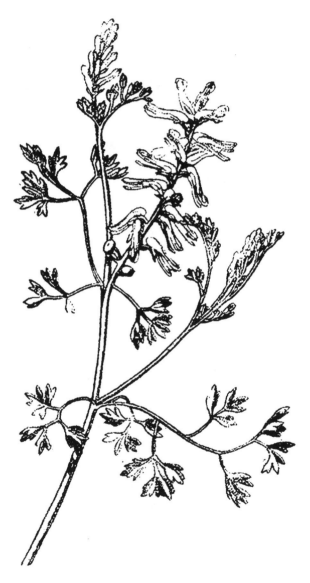

Botanical Description

Its whitish, blue-green colour gives it the appearance of smoke rising from the ground. Fumitory is a delicate annual, with a weak, trailing stem that often grows several feet. The leaves are much divided into numerous three-lobed segments, and both stem and leaves are perfectly smooth and hairless. It tends to climb, supporting itself by its twisted petioles. The whitish blue flowers grow in racemes (clusters) at the end of each stalk and opposite the leaves. Each flower has one petal that is swollen at the base into a pouch or spur. The rest of the flower is formed by oblong petals with dark coloured tips, which form a tube.

Healing Properties

Fumitory regulates the flow of bile. So if you are producing too much or too little bile, fumitory will normalise it. It prevents the formation of gallstones, so if you are prone to gallstones drink fumitory infusion. Since it is also antibiotic, a weak diuretic and laxative, it is used to purify the system and get rid of chronic eczema. In Germany, *Fumaria officinalis* is approved for "colicky pain affecting the gallbladder and biliary system, together with the gastrointestinal tract."

Chemical Constituents

Fumitory contains isoquinoline alkaloids, including protopine (fumarine), which is antihistamine, lowers blood pressure, strengthens heart rate and is sedative in small doses, whereas in larger doses it causes excitation and convulsions. It also contains flavonoids and the wound-healing chlorogenic acid.

Research

For a description of some of the research carried out on fumitory, see my book *The Healing Power of Celtic Plants*.

How to Use Fumitory

Make an infusion of fumitory, either dried or fresh to regulate your gall bladder if you are having problems digesting fats. It will calm your digestive system. Take the tincture to prevent gallstones.

Dosage

Herb 2–4g or by infusion three times a day.

Liquid extract (1:1 in 25% alcohol) 1–4ml three times a day.

Tincture (1:5 in 45% alcohol) 1–4ml three times a day.

Contraindications

Do not take fumitory if you are pregnant or breast feeding.

Chapter 9

Iris
Iris germanica

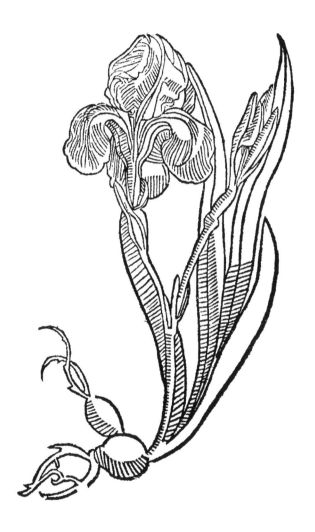

Some years ago I was in Florence at the beginning of May, visiting my son, who decided to take his students to visit the Iris Garden. We climbed the steep, narrow road up the hill to the garden on a beautiful, sunny day. We arrived at the top of the terraced garden, looking down on the city far below, the round dome of the Duomo rising out of the centre of Florence with its terracotta tiles glowing in the sunshine. As we stepped into the garden we were surrounded by irises of every shape and colour, as different from the original purple flowers, grown in fields in serried ranks for the perfume industry, as could be imagined.

The Iris garden in Florence was created in 1957 for the International Iris Competition by the Italian Iris Society. The competition is held every year and people continue to plant yet more exotic species.

Iris germanica is grown in Italy for the perfume industry. The dried rhizomes are known as orris root. When used for medicine they are known as *rhizome iridis*. When iris rhizomes are dried for less than two years and hydro-distilled this results in the production of retinoids, which smell like chocolate, or woody, leathery or hay-like. On the other hand when iris rhizomes are dried for three years, the fats and oils in them degrade, releasing fragrant compounds called irones, which smell like violets. The essential oil from three-year-old rhizomes is one of the most expensive and strengthens or enhances the fragrance of other aromatic herbs and prolongs their staying power.

The red lily was the symbol of Florence since the twelfth century. It was in fact originally a white iris on a red background until 1266, when the Guelphs, who defeated the Ghibellines, modified the symbol as a sign of their victory into a red iris (called a lily) on a white background.

Botanical Description

There are about three hundred species of iris with bulbs (or rhizomes) (thick, creeping underground stems.) The flowers consist of six petal-like floral segments, the more erect inner ones called standards and the drooping outer ones called falls. They have swordlike leaves and their tall stems grow up to 90cm with three to many flowers.

Healing Properties

Traditional healers have used the roots and rhizomes of many Iris species to treat coughs, colds, bronchitis and as an antispasmodic. They have used decoctions of the rhizomes to treat hormone-related diseases. The roots contain potent anti-cholinesterase, anti-cancer and anti-malarial compounds. Root decoctions loosen phlegm in the chest and lungs and act as expectorant, soothe sore throat and pacify coughing. Root decoctions also calm smooth muscle and control nausea. The root will relieve congestion and sluggishness in the liver. It stimulates the gall bladder to secrete bile, and the mouth to secrete saliva, which in turn stimulates both the appetite, the stomach and digestive system and speeds up elimination through the bowel. It is also decongestant, expectorant, diuretic, carminative, purgative and emmenagogue. Eclectic herbalists used it as cathartic, alterative, vermifuge and diuretic. Ellingwood, in his American Materia Medica said iris root stimulated the glandular system, but cautioned not to exceed the dose, since high doses were toxic.

Chemical Constituents

The main components are flavones, isoflavones, xanthones, quinones, terpenes, simple phenolics and plant steroids, such as beta-sitosterol, with multiple biological activities.

Research

For a description of the research carried out on Iris species see my book: *Healing Plants of Greek Myth*.

How to Use Iris

Make a decoction by boiling the powdered root 1–5 minutes in a cup of water or use a tincture of the root, and take to loosen phlegm in the chest and lungs and to act as expectorant, sooth sore throat and pacify coughing. Take for its laxative effect on the bowels, to relieve congestion and sluggishness in the liver, to stimulate the stomach and digestive system. Use together with other herbs to stimulate the lymphatic system and the kidneys to rid the body of toxins.

Use iris essential oil, diluted in a carrier oil in aromatherapy massage for its calming, relaxing effect.

Dosage

0.3–0.9g powdered root.

Tincture of orris root: Take 8–12 drops in juice or water, 3 times a day.

Shake well. Store in a cool dark place. Keep out of reach of children.

Contraindications

Pregnant and breast-feeding women should not take iris (orris) root. Some people are allergic to *rhizome iridis* though it seems to be safe for most people when taken by mouth as long as you don't exceed the dose. There are no known side effects if the root is carefully peeled and dried. However, the fresh plant juice or root can cause severe irritation of the mouth, stomach pain, vomiting, bloody diarrhoea and severe skin irritation. There isn't enough information to know if the dried *rhizome iridis* might be safe when applied directly to the skin.

Chapter 10

Ivy
Hedera helix

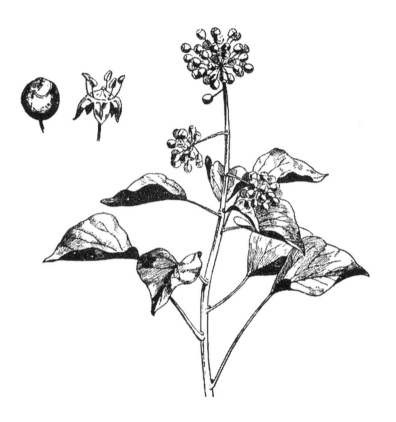

My sister and I shared a bedroom in the Georgian part of the farmhouse we grew up in, a farmhouse that had grown from an Elizabethan hall house into some kind of monstrosity with the addition of a large Georgian extension. Our lovely south facing bedroom had sash windows that looked out onto most of the garden and the Weald of Kent beyond, spread out in all its glory. The whole Georgian extension was covered in ivy, which provided nesting spaces for the hundreds of sparrows who woke us at dawn with their deafening chorus of twittering and tweeting.

Ivy has always been regarded as the emblem of fidelity. One of the early Councils of the Church forbade people to decorate their houses and churches with Ivy at Christmas because they considered it to be a pagan custom. This did not stop the practice. According to Mrs. Grieves, English taverns used to put an ivy bush over their doors as a sign of the excellence of their liquor: hence the saying 'Good wine needs no bush.'

Botanical Description

Ivy climbs using fibres which shoot out from every part of the stem with small disks at the end, which adapt themselves to the roughness of the bark or wall against which it is growing and to which it clings. These fibres burrow into every little crevice, becoming true roots. Ivy injures the trees it climbs up, sucking the juices out of them. When it reaches the top of the tree or wall it grows out in a bushy form and the leaves, instead of being five-lobed and angular as they are below, become ovate with entire margins.

Ivy only produces flowers when the branches rise above their support, the flowering branches being bushy and projecting a foot or two from the climbing stems with small, yellowish-green flowers at the end of every shoot. The flowers grow in clusters of nearly globular umbels with five broad, short petals and five stamens. They seldom open before the end of October and continue until late December. They have no scent but plenty of nectar. The berries ripen in the spring and provide food for many birds during severe winters. When ripe they are the size of a pea, black or deep purple, smooth and succulent and contain two to five seeds. Ivy is very hardy, tolerant of frost, smoke and pollution. It can live to a great age, its stems becoming woody and thick. Ivy which creeps over the ground never blossoms. The branches root into the soil.

Healing Properties

The leaves and berries of *Hedera helix* are anti-inflammatory, analgesic, immunological, anti-cancer, anti-mutagenic, antimicrobial, anti-parasitic, gastrointestinal, and antithrombin. According to the European Medicines Agency Committee on Herbal Medicinal Products: people have been using it to treat common colds, coughs, acute and chronic inflammatory bronchial disorders. According to Rashed in 2013 people have been using the leaves as analgesic and anti-inflammatory, taking the leaves and berries orally as an expectorant to treat cough and bronchitis. According to Chichiricco in 1980 people have applied ivy leaves to the skin to fight ringworm, scabies and to sooth cracks, grazes, chapped skin and insect bites. People used it to treat depression, as stimulant, narcotic and hallucinogenic depending on the amount that they drank.

Chemical Constituents

Ivy leaves contain unsaturated sterols, oils, tannins, phenolic compounds, saponins: hederacoside C, alpha-hederin, and hederagenin, terpenoids, glycosides, alkaloids, flavonoids, reducing sugars, volatile oil, vitamins: E, C, pro-vitamin A and carbohydrates.

Ivy berries contain triterpene saponins, polyacetylenes, fatty acids: petroselinic, oleic, cis-vaccenic, palmitoleic; and beta-lectins.

Research

In 2011 Wolf demonstrated in the laboratory that alpha hederin relaxed the muscles of the trachea. The European Pharmocopoea states that ivy leaf extract relaxes guinea pig bronchi when they are constricted. In 2012 Hocaoglu demonstrated that ivy extracts improved the breathing of asthmatic mice.

In 1980 Chichiricco carried out a double blind, placebo-controlled, randomised cross-over study on 30 children suffering from mild, persistent asthma. He gave ivy leaf extract to some of the children, in addition to their inhaled corticosteroid therapy and placebo plus inhaled corticosteroid therapy to the others. The children taking the ivy leaf extract improved significantly. In 2003 Hofmann reviewed the clinical trials that had been carried out on asthmatic children with ivy leaf extract. He found that it improved the breathing of children with chronic bronchial asthma.

In 2009 Fazio treated 9,657 patients suffering from bronchitis with ivy leaf syrup. 95% of the patients were improving after seven days. There were very few side effects. Antibiotics did not improve the symptoms but did cause adverse side effects. In 1942 Schmidt treated two hundred and sixty eight children suffering from bronchitis with either ivy herb extract syrup or ivy cough drops for 14 days. At the end of the study symptoms of rhinitis, cough and viscous mucus had greatly improved or completely cleared up in 93%, 94% and 97.7% respectively. All the children liked the cough drops and 99% liked the syrup.

In 2005 Buechi carried out a clinical trial on 62 patients suffering from coughs, with an ivy, thyme, aniseed and marshmallow root cough syrup. The main ingredient was ivy. 86% of them improved and 97% tolerated the cough syrup well. In 2011 Cwientzek carried out a double-blind randomised study on 590 patients with acute bronchitis. He treated the patients with two different ivy leaf extracts for seven days. Bronchitis decreased gradually in both groups taking the cough syrups and only 2.7% experienced any minor side effects. In 2006 Kemmerich carried out a double-blind, placebo controlled, multi centre study on 361 patients suffering from acute bronchitis. He found that a fluid extract of thyme and ivy leaves three times a day for eleven days was 47% effective compared to placebo. The group taking the extract were coughing half as much two days before the placebo group.

In 2013 Rai demonstrated that ivy extract was anti-inflammatory *in vivo*. The crude saponin extract had the most potent anti-inflammatory effect. In 2014 Rauf found that ivy extracts were analgesic and antioxidant in mice.

In 1996 Amara-Mokrane demonstrated *in vitro* that alpha hederin was anti-mutagenic. In 1990 Elias also found that alpha hederin was anti-mutagenic.

In 2016 Schulte-Michels demonstrated the anti-inflammatory effect of ivy leaf extract *in vitro*.

Thrombin plays an important part in the formation of blood clots, which are a necessary part of wound healing. It is only when blood clots form internally that people run the risk of stroke. In 2002 Medeiros demonstrated *in vitro* that ivy extracts had anti-thrombin effect. He isolated alpha amyrin and beta amyrin from the extract and tested them. He found that alpha amyrin had anti-thrombin effect. Then he isolated stigmasterol from the extract and found that this also had anti-thrombin effect.

How to Use Ivy

Take an ivy tincture or extract to ease a cough, bronchitis or asthma.

You could make a cough mixture with ivy, thyme and marshmallow root tinctures, or you could make a tea with ivy leaves. You could make a poultice by mixing fresh ivy leaves with linseed meal and spreading it on a cloth on the sick person's chest. They would have to stay lying on their back while the poultice worked its effect. This might be difficult if the patient was coughing hard.

Dosage

Tincture (in daily doses): 250–420mg for adult, 150–210mg for children 4–12 years,

50–150mg for children 1–4 years, 20–50mg for children 0–1 year.

Alcohol-free preparations: 300–945mg for adults; 200–630mg for children 4–12 years; 150–300mg for children 1–4 years; 50–200mg for children 0–1 year.

Make a tea by adding 1 heaped teaspoonful (0.3–0.8g) of dried leaves to 250ml of boiling water and steeping for 10 minutes. Take 1–3 times daily, sweetened if desired.

Contraindications

Be careful not to take more than the recommended dose.

Do not take ivy if you are pregnant or lactating. Patients with gastritis or gastric ulcer should avoid ivy. Be careful with children under six years old.

Ivy extract has been tested for toxicity on mice and rats and even high doses did not kill them, though they did cause diarrhoea. Patients who took ivy extracts did not suffer any serious side effects, though a few did suffer from diarrhoea, stomach ache, nausea and vomiting, skin allergy, dry mouth, anorexia, anxiety headache and drowsiness. The fresh leaves, however, can cause contact dermatitis. Some people are allergic to ivy and should wear protective clothing if they have to work with it.

Chapter 11

Juniper
Juniperus communis

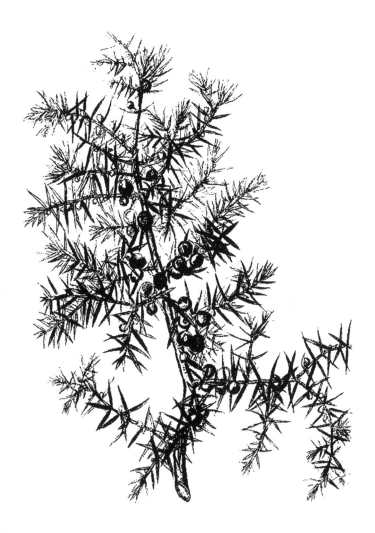

The cows who roam the common near where I live, avoid the prickly little juniper bushes that cling to the steep slopes, their berries ripening slowly.

People have been distilling juniper berries for centuries to extract the essential oil. Commercially juniper berries are used to flavour teas, beers, liqueurs (Ginepro) alcoholic bitters and gin. The word gin may be a shortened form of the Dutch genever, which is derived from the Latin *juniperus*, or it may be derived from the term Holland's Geneva, as the Dutch-invented drink was first known.

Botanical Description

Juniper is a member of the Cypress family: the Cupressaceae, and can grow as a dense, evergreen shrub, creeping along the ground, or a small tree, up to 600cm high. It has dark green to blue green pointed leaves and blue or reddish berries a quarter to half an inch wide. Juniper berries take two or three years to ripen, so that there are blue and green berries on the same plant.

Parts Used

The berries.

Healing Properties

Juniper is anti-rheumatic, antiseptic, carminative, diuretic and stomachic. Juniper oil is astringent, anti-inflammatory and antiseptic. According to Mrs. Grieve, Juniper oil is good for indigestion, flatulence, heartburn, bloating, loss of appetite, gastrointestinal infections, intestinal worms and diseases of the kidney and bladder.

Chemical Constituents

Juniper berries and needles contain volatile oil. The needle oil consists mainly of sabinene (40.7%), α-pinene (12.5%) and terpinen-4-ol (12.3%) and the berry oil includes sabinene (36.8%), alpha-pinene (20%), limonene (10.6%), germacrene D (8.2%) and myrcene (4.8%). Juniper berries also contain neolignans, flavonoid glycosides, biflavonyls, sequiterpenes, diterpenes and fatty acids.

Research

There have been some *in vitro* and animal studies on juniper but no one has yet carried out any human clinical studies. For a full account of the research that has been carried out on Juniper, see my book: *Healing Plants of the Celtic Druids*.

How to Use Juniper

Pick the berries when they are ripe and dry them. Juniper is very powerful medicine, should be used with great care and never long term. It inhibits the formation of inflammatory prostaglandins. Herbalists combine it with other herbs as a diuretic to treat urinary problems, although the German Commission E does not approve juniper for kidney and bladder complaints. It does, however, approve aqueous infusions and decoctions of juniper dried fruit, alcoholic extracts, wine extracts or essential oil to relieve indigestion or disturbed digestion. In 2008 Health Canada recommended juniper fruit as a diuretic and urinary tract antiseptic to help relieve benign urinary tract infections.

In addition juniper berries help clear congestion and are often included in cold remedies to improve breathing.

Make an infusion by pouring a pint of boiling water over 30g of berries and leaving to steep. Take cupfuls to detoxify the body and help allay the symptoms of gout and rheumatoid arthritis, to relieve digestive disturbances such as flatulent dyspepsia, to aid digestion and stimulate your appetite.

Massage with the diluted essential oil to ease neuralgia, sciatica and rheumatic pains. Dilute juniper oil in a carrier oil to cleanse and tone the skin in cases of skin inflammations such as acne and eczema. Juniper oil has a strengthening, tonic effect on the nerves. Inhale the essential oil of juniper to treat bronchitis.

Dosage

1:1 liquid extract with 25% ethanol: 0.1ml.

1:5 tincture with 45% ethanol: 0.1ml.

20 to 100mg of the essential oil diluted in a carrier oil for massage.

Contraindications

Juniper is the most active but also the most potentially toxic of the volatile-oil-containing berries used to treat infections of the urinary tract. Use Juniper with great care and do not take on a regular basis. Do not use during pregnancy or lactation or in cases of kidney disease. Overdose can cause convulsions and damage the kidneys. Use juniper berry essential oils sparingly. Some people are allergic to juniper.

Chapter 12

Laurel or Bay
Laurus nobilis

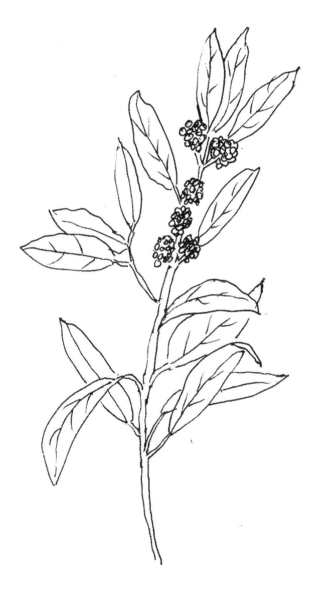

The name Lorenzo (*Laurentius* in Latin) is similar to the word lauro or laurel, with its many classical associations. Florentine poets celebrated this link in their verses honouring Lorenzo the Magnificent. Angelo Poliziano, for example, wrote these lines:

> And you well-born Laurel, under whose veil
> Florence rests happily in peace
> Fearing neither the wind nor the threat of the sky.

It would seem that he was referring to Lorenzo's magnificent actions which saved Florence from invasion, for which, according to Roman tradition, he should be crowned with laurels.

Botanical Description

The laurel or sweet bay is a small tree, 2–15m tall, with olive-green or reddish smooth bark. The luxurious evergreen leaves with short stalks, grow alternately and are lanceolate with smooth, wavy margins. They are thick, smooth and shining dark green. Laurel produces male and female flowers, which are small, yellow, 4-lobed and grow in small clusters; the male has 8–12 stamens and the female 2–4 staminodes. The fruit is 1–1.5cm, ovoid, and purplish black when ripe. It grows well under the shade of other trees. People cook with the aromatic leaves.

Healing Properties

The leaves are antiseptic, aromatic, astringent, digestive, diuretic, anti-parasitic and stimulant. They relieve flatulence. If you boil them up and drink the resultant tea when suffering from a cold they will bring out a sweat and rid the body of toxins, helping you to recover more quickly. In large doses they are emetic, emmenagogue and narcotic. They are used traditionally to treat bronchitis, influenza and to aid digestion. They have a tonic effect, stimulating the appetite and the secretion of digestive juices. The fruit is narcotic and people used it as an emmenagogue (a euphemism for a substance which produces an abortion).

Chemical Constituents

Lauris nobilis contains sesquiterpene lactones such as 10-epigazaniolide, gazaniolide, spirafolide, costunolide, reynosin, santamarine; flavonoid glycosides and essential oil. The essential oil contains a multitude of compounds such as: cineole, α-terpinyl acetate, terpinene-4-ol, alpha-pinene, beta-pinene, p-cymene and linalool acetate.

Research

Bay laurel has wound healing, nerve-protective, antioxidant, anti-ulcer, anti-convulsant, anti-mutagenic, anti-viral, anti-cholinergic, anti-bacterial and anti-fungal properties. For a full description of the research which has been carried out on laurel please see my book: *Healing Plants of Greek Myth*. People have been cooking with bay leaves and using them as medicine for thousands of years. It is easy to grow a small bay tree, either in a pot on a balcony or planted in your garden.

How to Use Laurel

Make a tea with 2 bay leaves and a pint of boiled water. Leave to steep for five minutes and drink to sooth a sore throat, cough, bronchitis. You can add ginger, honey, lemon.

Drink a bay leaf tea at bedtime to help you sleep.

Grind up 10–20 bay leaves and add them to your bath, to calm the mind and body. Their anti-inflammatory, antibacterial and anti-fatigue properties will relax aching muscles and joints.

When cooking with bay leaves be sure to remove them before eating.

Contraindications

Don't use bay leaves for at least two weeks before surgery because they might slow down the central nervous system too much during anaesthesia. People taking medications for high blood sugar should avoid bay leaf.

Chapter 13

Lemon
Citrus limon

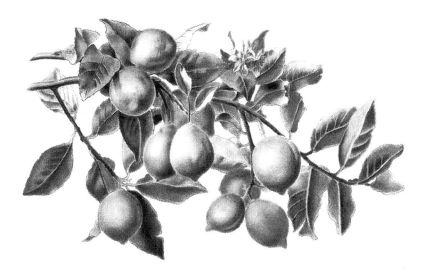

The first citrus trees appeared about eight million years ago in the southeast foothills of the Himalayas, including the eastern area of Assam, northern Myanmar and western Yunnan, before spreading throughout southeast Asia. About four million years ago they spread to the rest of the world. Today's citrus fruits were evolving for millions of years, followed by thousands of years of human plant breeding. Around 400 CE they were planted in orchards in Moorish Spain, according to McGee in 2004. It was used as an ornamental plant in early Islamic gardens according to Julia Morton in 1987. The first substantial cultivation of lemons in Europe began in Genoa in the middle of the 15th century. In Renaissance Florence citrus trees were still rare and considered exotic. Cosimo I de' Medici planted various species in his gardens.

Botanical Description

The lemon is a small evergreen tree or spreading bush of the Rutaceae family, 3–6m high with oval leaves which have a reddish tint when young, later turning green. The flowers are solitary or in small clusters in the axils of the leaves, reddish tinted buds turn white when open. Lemon flowers are perfumed. The fruit is oval, with a broad, low, apical nipple and forms 8–10 segments. The outer rind or peel is yellow and dotted with oil glands. The white, spongy, inner part of the peel is the mesocarp and the chief source of commercial pectin. The seeds are small, ovoid, pointed.

Healing Properties

The juice and the peel of lemons are anti-inflammatory, anti-bacterial, anti-fungal, help the liver to regenerate and protect the heart. The essential oil of lemon peel has been used since the 18th century to produce 'Eau de Cologne' and is used to mask unpleasant tastes in pharmaceutical preparations and as a preserving agent. People use it in aromatherapy to calm the patient, relax muscles and to treat numerous conditions, such as high blood pressure, neurosis, anxiety, varicose veins, arthritis, rheumatism and menopausal symptoms. If you put a drop of lemon on your tongue when you've lost your sense of taste, it stimulates the taste mechanisms in the tongue.

Chemical Constituents

Lemon skin contains an essential oil, which is considered a pharmacopeial raw material, cited in the European Pharmacopaeia, the American Pharmacopoeia and the Ayurvedic Pharmacopoeia in India. This essential oil is rich in bioactive monoterpenoids, such as D-limonene, beta-pinene and gamma-terpinene. Lemons contain flavonoids: diosmin, hesperidin, limocitrin, eriodictyol, hesperetin, naringin;

flavones: apigenin, diosmin; flavonols: quercetin; and phenolic acids: ferric, synaptic, p-hydoxybenzoic acids.

Research

In 2015 Raimondo isolated nano vesicles from lemon juice and demonstrated that they inhibited cancer cells from growing and caused them to die *in vitro*. Nano vesicles also suppressed leukaemia tumour growth *in vivo*. In the same year, Parhiz reviewed the research that demonstrated the antioxidant and anti-inflammatory activity of the lemon flavonoids, hesperidin and hesperetin. In 2016 Otang demonstrated that lemon peel extracts were effective against bacteria and had antioxidant effect so it made sense that the Xhosa tribe of Amathole District, Eastern Cape, South Africa were using lemon peel to treat skin diseases. In 2013 Hamdan demonstrated that lemon essential oil ingredients, D-limonene, beta-pinene and citral were anti-fungal *in vitro*. In 2016 Aboelhadid demonstrated that lemon essential oil diluted in water killed parasitic mites infecting rabbits. In 2013 Tsujiyama demonstrated that lemon peel extracts inhibited histamine release and suppressed inflammation *in vivo*. In 2007 Bhavsar demonstrated that a lemon extract prevented liver damage in rats and helped damaged liver to regenerate. In 2013 Mohanapriya gave lemon peel extract to diabetic rats and demonstrated that their blood glucose levels and wound healing time fell and they had an increase in tissue growth rate, collagen sysnthesis and protein levels. In 2012 Murali demonstrated an anti-diabetic effect, comparable with that of glibenclamide, of d-limonene in diabetic rats. Millet showed in 2014 that D-limonene lowers LDL-cholesterol, prevents the accumulation of fats and lowers blood sugar levels in rats. He also demonstrated that D-limonene settles the stomach, neutralises stomach acids and relieves gastric reflux. In 2013 Lima demonstrated that D-limonene had a calming effect on mice. It also had a painkilling effect.

Murali in 2012 mentioned a study which demonstrated that lemon juice, when combined with exercise, lowered blood pressure in a group of Japanese middle-aged women. It would be interesting to see whether the lemon juice without the exercise had a comparable effect.

Conclusions

I'm sure you already use lemons in cooking and drinks. Use slithers of the peel as well, or grate the peel with a very fine grater. Add the juice of a lemon to water, either hot or cold for a refreshing, low-calorie drink, rich in vitamin C.

Contraindications

Lemon juice and essential oil should not be used in high concentrations in baths or directly on the skin. The essential oil should always be diluted in a carrier oil. Some people are allergic to D-limonene, which is in the essential oil. If you use cosmetics containing lemon peel essential oil you must avoid the sun because it contains photosensitising compounds.

Chapter 14

Myrtle
Myrtus communis

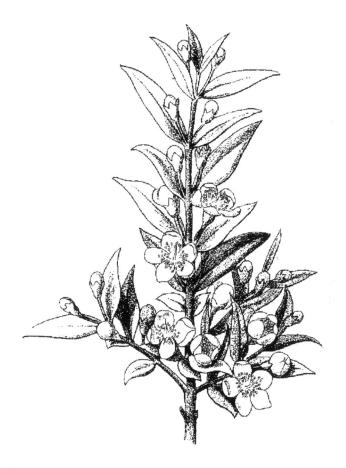

The Unani System of Medicine has been using common myrtle since the time of the ancient Greeks. Unani healers use the berries, leaves and essential oil for gastric ulcer, diarrhoea, dysentery, vomiting, rheumatism, haemorrhages, sinusitis and leucorrhoea (a whitish or yellowish discharge of mucus from the vagina).

Botanical Description

Myrtle has an upright stem, 2.4–3m high, its branches form a close full head, thickly covered with evergreen leaves. Its stem is branched and the dark green leaves are thick, stiff, glossy, smooth, hairless, ovate to lanceolate and grow opposite each other in pairs, or whorled. They are aromatic, with smooth edges and 2.5–3.8cm long, without glands on the blade of the leaf. Myrtle has stiff white flowers about 2cm diameter that grow from an axil on slender stalks, with yellow anthers. The petals are pure white with glands and somewhat hairy edges. They give off a sweet fragrant smell. The berries are 0.7–1.2cm, about the size of a pea, round or ovoid-ellipsoid, blue-black or white with hard kidney shaped seeds. They start off pale green, then turn deep red and finally become dark indigo when fully mature. They are bitter when unripe, sweet when ripe.

Healing Properties

The leaves are aromatic, balsamic, tonic, astringent, antiseptic, laxative, analgesic and lower blood sugar and stop blood flow from wounds. The root is anti-bacterial according to Agarwal in 1986. People use myrtle to treat urinary infections, digestive problems, bronchial congestion, and dry coughs. They use it externally to treat wounds, gum infections and haemorrhoids. Essential oil of myrtle leaves is antiseptic and is used to treat acne and rheumatism.

The fruit is antiseptic, carminative, astringent and emmenagogue, according to Nadkarni in 1989; and used to treat dysentery, diarrhoea, haemorrhoids and ulcers. It is soothing and analgesic, and stops the flow of blood from wounds, according to Baitar in 1999. In 1920 Ghani stated that the berries were a tonic for the heart, stomach and brain and were diuretic and would break up kidney stones and stop vomiting. They are anti-inflammatory and protect the kidneys, according to Hakeem in 1895.

Chemical Constituents

The plant contains a wide range of biologically active compounds such as tannins, flavonoids, coumarins, fixed oil, sugars, citric acid, malic acid and antioxidants as well as high quantities of vitamins and essential oil. Almost all the volatile compounds in the essential oil are terpenes and terpene alcohols: 1,8-cineole, alpha-pinene, myrtenyl acetate, limonene, linalool and alpha-terpinolene. The essential oil is extracted from the leaves, branches, fruits and flowers through steam distillation. The main active compounds in myrtle leaves are polyphenols, Myrtucommulone (MC) and semi-myrtucommulone (S-MC), unique compounds.

The major compounds in the berries are phenolic compounds, flavonoids and anthocyanins. They contain citric acid, malic acid, resin, tannin, fixed oil and 14 fatty acids, including oleic (67.07%) palmitic (10.24%) and stearic acid (8.19%.) The seeds contain 12–15% fatty oil consisting of glycerides of oleic, linoleic, myristic, palmitic, linolenic and lauric acid. The roots contain tannins, alkaloids, glycosides, reducing sugars, fixed oil, gallic acids, phenolic acids, quercetin and patuletin.

Research

Several scientists have demonstrated that myrtle extract is anti-bacterial, anti-fungal, anti-inflammatory, antioxidant, free radical scavenging, anti-diabetic and anti-cancer. Clinical trials have demonstrated that myrtle improves mouth ulcers, athletic performance and bacterial vaginosis. For a full description of this scientific research see my book: *Healing Plants of Greek Myth*.

Although the myrtle plant has so many active constituents and such promising therapeutic possibilities, there have been few clinical trials. It would appear that scientists are more interested in isolating compounds with interesting activity which could be developed by the pharmaceutical industry.

How to Use Myrtle

Use myrtle essential oil in a vaporiser to ease chronic bronchial and lung conditions, to help expel phlegm from the lungs and bronchi, to aid sleep. Use it to help people suffering from withdrawal from addiction to drugs and to soothe and ease self destructive behaviour and feelings of anger, fear, greed and envy.

Mix with a carrier oil and use in aromatherapy to treat physical exhaustion, anxiety, insomnia, depression, nervous tension and stress. Blend a few drops into a cream to correct over-dry or over oily skin and to eradicate acne. Make an ointment with witch hazel, cypress essential oil and myrtle essential oil for an astringent effect on piles.

Make a tea with myrtle leaves to treat bronchial congestion and dry cough. Use as a vaginal wash to treat bacterial and yeast infections.

Chapter 15

Mustard
Brassica nigra

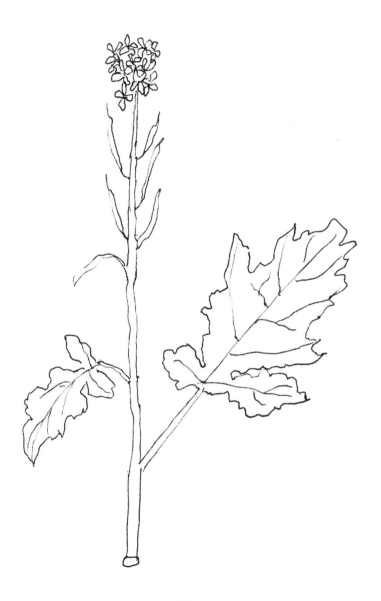

There are approximately forty different species of mustard plant. Three different types are generally used to make the mustard condiment. Black mustard (*Brassica nigra*) is the most pungent. White mustard (*Brassica alba*) is the mildest and is used to make traditional American yellow mustard. Brown mustard (*Brassica juncea*) is dark yellow, has a pungent taste, and is used to make Dijon mustard.

Botanical Description

Mustard, a member of the Brassica family, is an annual plant growing up to 200cm, branching from the middle or from near the base. Mustard plants have alternate leaves with ruffled margins and produce small, yellow four-petaled flowers. The lower leaves are hairy and have 1–3 pairs of pointed lateral lobes and a much larger lobe at the end. The upper leaves are hairless. The flowers have 7–13mm long yellow petals. The seed capsule is 8–30mm long and 1.5–4.5mm wide with a slender, seedless beak.

Healing Properties

Mustard flour has preservative, antioxidant, anti-cancer, anti-bacterial, anti-fungal and anti-helminthic properties. It protects against kidney and liver toxicity and has been used in diabetes treatment. Black mustards are also used in cardiovascular and neurological disorders. Mustard is decongestant. It helps to clear mucus from the throat and bronchi. Inhaling the steam of heated mustard seeds or gargling with mustard tea, helps to expel mucus from the throat and lungs. Yellow mustard is rich in monounsaturated and polyunsaturated fats that help in balancing cholesterol levels. Yellow mustard is an effective home remedy for bad breath. It is loaded with beta-carotene, protein, iron and calcium which help to promote hair growth and keep your hair healthy.

Chemical Constituents

Brassica nigra contains glycosinolates which are broken down by enzyme tyrosinase, in the presence of water, transforming them into allyl isothiocyanate. Mustard seed oil contains 90% allyl isothiocyanate and terpenes, which have anti-inflammatory properties and are the primary constituents of mustard essential oil. The seeds also contain about 30% proteins, 27% fixed oil, inosite, lecithin, albumins, mucilage, flavonoids and other phenolic compounds and a variety of minerals, including iron, magnesium, zinc, calcium, and phosphorus.

Mustard greens are nutrient dense and contain high amounts of vitamins, such as vitamins A, K, and C, and minerals, such as calcium.

Research

In 2015 Tripathi demonstrated that allyl isothiocyanate in mustard seeds killed lung cancer cells *in vitro*. In 2010 Bhattacharya inhibited bladder cancer growth with isothiocyanate-rich mustard seed powder. In 2014 Xie demonstrated that mustard seeds suppressed colon cancers in mice and in 2008 Chou showed that it suppressed colorectal cancers in rats. In 2015 Nauman found that mustard extracts protected human liver cells, colorectal cells, brain cells, breast cancer cells.

Isothiocyanates may also decrease multi-drug resistance in human cancer cell lines and inhibit the removal of cancer-treating drugs from cells, which enhances the effect of chemotherapy treatment.

In 2002 Tseng found that isothiocyanates increased the accumulation of anti-cancer drugs in multi-drug resistant cancer cells by inhibiting the removal of these drugs from the cancer cells.

Both mustard leaves and seeds can lower blood glucose in animals with type two diabetes. In 2003 Kim demonstrated *in vitro* and *in vivo* that mustard leaf extract reduced the oxidation of fats, reduced free radicals and lessened the damage caused by oxidative stress. Researchers speculated that mustard enhances the conversion of glucose into pyruvate, releasing free high-energy and decreases the storage of glycogen in the body's tissues. In 2004 Yadav found that mustard powder decreased blood glucose, insulin, and cholesterol levels in rats fed a high-fructose diet. He concluded that mustard may delay or prevent the onset of diabetes in addition to mitigating its effects.

Cardiovascular disease (CVD) is often studied together with diabetes, as individuals with diabetes tend to suffer from CVD. In 2012 John examined the effects of two doses of mustard seed powder on serum cholesterol and triglycerides in diabetic rats. He found that 8g/kg of body weight lowered both. He suggested that mustard might mimic or enhance the effectiveness of insulin, lowering the amount patients would need to take.

There are often neurological complications associated with diabetes. In 2013 Thakur found that a mustard extract improved brain chemistry and cognitive function in rats, and speculated that neurological problems could be improved by eating mustard or taking supplements. He also found that mustard compensated for low levels of neurotransmitters: norepinephrine, serotonin and dopamine in rat brains. This resulted in improvement of feelings of helplessness and despair, as well as impaired locomotion (though it is hard to imagine how he could tell that the rats were feeling despair!)

Mustard is anti-bacterial and anti-viral and protects cells from the damage caused by microbes and viruses. In 2012 Rajamurugan found that mustard extract protected rats with hepatitis from liver and kidney damage. He thought that anti-inflammatory compounds, such as terpenes, in mustard were responsible for this protective action.

Mustard is also antifungal. In 2015 Mejía-Garibay demonstrated that mustard essential oil inhibited several types of fungi and prevented further growth.

How to Use Laurel

To make a strong, pungent mustard, mix the flour with room temperature water. To produce a milder flavour mix the mustard flour with vinegar. To make a mustard plaster make a paste by mixing ground black mustard seed with warm water then pack the paste in cloth and apply the cloth directly to the skin. People use this preparation to treat pneumonia and pleurisy. But pneumonia and pleurisy are life-threatening conditions so you should see a doctor rather than self-medicating. You could use a mustard plaster to treat pain and swelling, arthritis and lower back pain but the patient would have to lie on their front with the plaster on their back. Not many people would want to do this. A mustard bath for aching feet is a more viable option. Mustard is decongestant. It helps to clear mucus from the throat and bronchi. Inhale the steam of heated mustard seeds or gargle with mustard tea, to expel mucus from the throat and lungs.

Contraindications

Eating normal amounts of mustard as a condiment is safe but eating large amounts of black mustard seed can damage the throat and cause other serious side effects including heart failure, diarrhoea, drowsiness, breathing difficulties, coma, and death. Mustard seed oil is not recognised as safe in the United States, Canada, and European Union due to its high erucic acid content. It can be highly irritable to the skin and mucous membranes and can cause skin blisters and skin damage.

Pregnant and breast-feeding women shouldn't use mustard. Do not use mustard if you are diabetic. High levels of vitamin K in mustard leaves could interact with certain blood-thinning medications such as warfarin, due to vitamin K's blood-coagulating properties. The vitamin K content could also be a concern to individuals with existing untreated thyroid issues or an iodine deficiency. Due to the high oxalate content of the leaves, people who suffer from oxalate-containing kidney stones should not eat mustard leaves.

Chapter 16

Olive
Olea europea

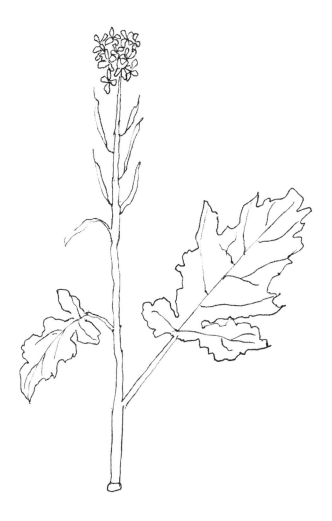

Years ago, when I lived in Italy, I had an olive grove on a steep, terraced hillside. Every year in November my sister and I went to pick the olives, spreading out nets under the trees and scrambling about on the icy branches combing the olives off so that they fell in a pattering rain onto the nets below. When we had picked the whole crop we took the bags of olives to the press, an old-fashioned cold press where the olives were ground into a paste with water, then spread onto round mats which were stacked one above the other on a long metal pole, above which the press loomed. After pressing, the resultant dirty looking mixture was whirled round in a centrifuge to separate out the oil. People who brought their olives to be pressed came with slices of bread which they held under the tap from which the freshly pressed oil dripped, so that they could taste it, green, pungent and full of healing properties.

In 2023 Francesca Gorini wrote an article for the Olive Oil times about the air-cleaning properties of olive trees. VegPM, she explained, was a research project coordinated by the University of Florence, which aimed to identify the most suitable plants for combating air pollution caused by particulate matter (minute particles in the air.) The project collected data from Lucca, Porcari, Capannori and Altopascio, all affected by high levels of fine particles, mostly caused by road traffic. Heating systems, waste management and agriculture also contributed to the problem. Particles can cause severe respiratory diseases, especially in children and the elderly. Federico Martinelli, associate professor of Genetics at the department of biology of the university of Florence said:

> As a first step, we made an extensive screening of the available species capable of absorbing/trapping more particles, heavy metals and ozone…By integrating the values recorded by the monitoring centres with the particulate accumulated in the leaves of each species analysed, we were able to rank the species with the highest PM deposition values.

They found that olive trees, in particular could accumulate large amounts of pollution. They could also tolerate drought and salinity.

The *spezeria* in Renaissance Florence did not list olive oil as one of the products it sold. Everyone had their own olive oil, from relatives in the countryside or simply bought from a shop. However, it would have been one of the oils the *spezeria* would have used to make their infused oils and unguents. It was so common an ingredient that they did not have need to mention it.

Botanical Description

Olea europaea is a small, evergreen tree which can grow up to 20m high, with pale grey bark, thin branches with opposite branchlets and shortly stalked, opposite, lanceolate, pointed, smooth leaves, pale green above and silvery below. It has numerous small, creamy white flowers. The fruit is an ovoid drupe. I think everyone knows what an olive looks like.

Healing Properties

In traditional medicine, olive leaves are used to fight colds, flu, yeast infections, viral infections, shingles and herpes. Olive leaves are used to support the heart, to treat high blood pressure, gout, arteriosclerosis and rheumatism. *Olea europaea* leaves bring down blood pressure and high temperature, stimulate the production of bile, are diuretic, laxative, skin cleanser, and are used to treat urinary infections, gallstones, bronchial asthma and diarrhoea.

Chemical constituents

Olive leaves contain oleuropein, a secoiridoid glucoside with a multitude of useful properties. Two of its by-products are also present in the rest of the olive plant: demethyl-oleuropein and the oleoside methyl ester. These two compounds increase in the olives as they ripen, while the quantity of oleuropein decreases. The leaves also contain glycosides, flavonoids, poly-unsaturated fatty acids and the anti-viral calcium elenolate. Olives also contain ligstroside, oleuroside, cornoside and esters of tyrosol and hydroxyl-tyrosol.

Research

Many scientists have carried out research to prove that olive is antioxidant, anti-viral, anti-microbial, anti-diabetic and has potential for use for cardiovascular disorders. Clinical studies have consistently demonstrated that the people who live on a Mediterranean diet, rich in olive oil, fruits, vegetables and grains, have a lower than average risk of coronary heart disease, according to Kushi in 1995. For a full description of this research see my book: *Healing Plants of Greek Myth*. Here are just a few of the clinical trials that have been carried out.

High blood pressure is a harmful disease that develops unnoticed over time. Ideally it should be diagnosed early and the patient should make lifestyle changes rather than taking harmful drugs. In 1949 Capretti and Bonaconza gave human adult patients 5ml of an olive leaf infusion or 3ml of an olive leaf decoction to drink once daily for 20–25 days. They noticed a diuretic effect. In 2008 Perrinjaquet-Moccetti and team carried out an open study on 40 monozygotic twins with borderline high blood pressure. They gave 500 or 1000mg/day of olive leaf extract (EFLA R 943), to each pair of twins in one group for 8 weeks or advice on a favourable lifestyle to another group of twins. Blood pressure decreased significantly within pairs, depending on the dose of olive leaf extract.

In 2011 Susalit carried out a double-blind, randomised, parallel and active-controlled clinical study to find out whether an olive leaf extract (EFLA R 943) would lower blood pressure, in patients with stage 1 high blood pressure. They gave half the patients 500mg of olive leaf extract orally twice daily for 8 weeks. They gave the control 12.5mg Captopril twice daily.

After 8 weeks of treatment, blood pressure of both groups fell. Triglycerides levels also fell in the group who took the olive leaf extract but not in the Captopril group. The olive leaf extract contained 18–26% (m/m) oleuropein, 30–40% (m/m) polyphenols as well as verbascoside and luteolin-7-glucoside.

In 2012 Weinstein and team carried out a controlled clinical trial with 79 adults with type 2 diabetes. They gave half the patients a 500mg olive leaf extract tablet per day and placebo to the other half for 14 weeks. The blood sugar and insulin of the subjects treated with olive leaf extract fell.

How to Use Olive Leaf

The healing properties of olive leaves are well-known. The European Medicine Authority say that since people have been using it for a long time, they can allow its use to promote water elimination through the kidneys. They do not recommend it for anything else. Take olive leaf to normalise blood pressure. If your blood pressure is abnormally high you should consult a doctor but if it is only slightly raised you could take olive leaf to lower it, in addition to taking plenty of exercise and cutting down on salt. Take olive leaf to stimulate your immune system, as a skin cleanser, to treat urinary infections, gallstones, bronchial asthma and diarrhoea.

Many of the healing compounds in the leaves are also present in the oil, in lesser quantities. Make sure that you obtain cold pressed organic olive oil for the maximum health benefit. In Mediterranean countries people drizzle olive oil onto salads, soups, cooked vegetables, rice, pasta and many other dishes, relishing the taste of it.

Dosage

Liquid olive leaf tincture: 30–50 drops, 3 times daily.

Hard capsules (containing 275mg powder each) 3–5 times daily.

Because formulations and products can vary, follow your doctor's recommendation and manufacturer's guidelines to ensure you take a safe but effective amount.

Contraindications

People with low blood pressure or taking blood pressure lowering medications should not take olive leaf extract. Anyone with hypoglycaemia or taking insulin should not take olive leaf extract. Olive leaf may conflict with some antibiotics.

Chapter 17

Orpine
Sedum telephium or *Hylotelephium telephium*

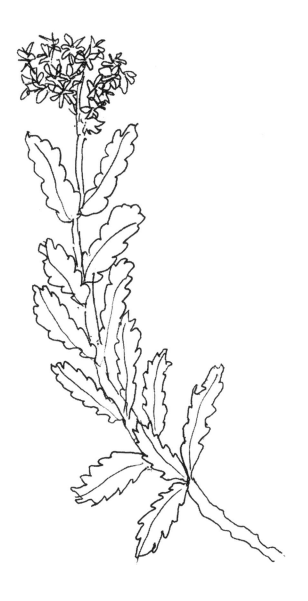

I saw orpine growing in the herb garden of the Santa Maria Nuova hospital, where it had been grown for the *spezeria* since the herb garden was first planted, way before the Renaissance.

Dr Sergio Balatri said:

On the fifth October 1978 I was on call at the San Giovanni di Dio Hospital in Borgo Ognissanti, Florence. Antonio, a young cobbler entered the Emergency ward with a flesh wound on his thumb which was not healing. He'd been to another hospital where they'd prescribed an antibiotic because the bone was infected and they'd told him that if it didn't heal they'd have to amputate. He decided to seek a second opinion and came to San Giovanni di Dio. As soon as I saw him, I don't know why but the Madonna's herb that my mother had shown me came to mind. I found it in Via Cassia from Roberto Benoni. He asked me whether this was the plant that one peels and applies to wounds. I sent Antonio to buy the herb which he brought back to me. I peeled a leaf and put it on the wound and told him to continue to do this every day. After ten days it had healed. I told the pharmacists in the hospital. One of them, Franco Vincieri was interested in plants and with the chemist Massimo Bambagiotti, had organised a phytochemical laboratory in the Pharmacy Faculty in Florence. He encouraged me to study plants and taught me the scientific name: *Sedum telephium*.

I began to study at the faculty of Natural Sciences where I discovered the long abandoned story of Plant Medicine. In the spring and summer of 1979 the leaves of the Madonna herb grew and my studies progressed. I went in search of the leaves in gardens and windowsills. At this time I'd started to treat gluteus abscesses with finely chopped *Sedum* leaves, to the amusement of my colleagues. But the abscesses healed.

That year I thought of freezing some leaves for the winter. Freezing and thawing the leaf, in addition to facilitating the removal of the cuticle from the lower epidermis, causes the breakdown of the parenchyma cells, making the active ingredients available to spread onto the surface one wants to treat. I cured a boil on the nose with some thawed out frozen leaves and published a paper in the Bollettino della Società in 1981.

In 1997 I began to collaborate with Daniela Giachetti at the University of Siena. In 2006 Sergio Boncinelli from the University of Florence Anaesthesia department organised a seminar on the interaction between plants and anaesthetic drugs and invited me to talk about the Madonna herb. I met Franco Bettiol, specialist in pharmaceutical preparations and proposed making a gel from the juice of Sedum. The Kos company made a gel which is now available to buy. Marina Ziche and Lucia Morbidelli demonstrated that Sedum modulates inflammation. Prof Marco Biagi is continuing to study this plant family.

Balatri is now retired but continues to study and use Sedum. Scientists at the University of Florence and Siena continued to experiment with *Sedum* and identified flavonoids and polysaccharides from the leaves with pharmacological activity.

According to Guarrere in 2006 and Biagi in 2013 *Sedum telephium* has been used traditionally throughout Italy for centuries and is mentioned in various ancient medical texts. According to Vitalini in 2015 people have been using it to treat insect bites, burns, corns, ulcers, warts, abscesses and wounds. People apply the fresh leaves to wounds and use the expressed juice to treat scars. In modern times herbal medicine doctors have been using *Sedum telephium* to treat serious emergency cases such as open wounds and second and third degree burns, or for major traumatic events such as broken bones, according to Balatri in 2013.

Botanical Description

The Sedum genus contains around 600 species of leaf succulents known as stonecrops and grows throughout the Northern Hemisphere. *Sedum telephium* is a clump-forming, deciduous perennial with erect, pale green stems bearing fleshy, grey-green leaves. It produces small, dark pink, star-shaped flowers in dense clusters in late summer and early autumn.

Healing Properties

Sedum telephium is anti-bacterial, anti-inflammatory, anti-oxidant and wound-healing. Applying the leaves to a wound keeps it free of infection, prevents free radical damage, calms inflammation, and promotes wound healing. The leaves, gel or extract can be used to treat wounds, ulcers, whitlows, abscesses, dermatitis, burns and also to draw out foreign bodies (splinters etc.) that are embedded in the skin.

Chemical Constituents

The main chemical constituents of the fresh juice of *Sedum telephium* are polyphenols and more than 5% soluble polysaccharides, according to Bonina in 2000. *Sedum telephium* contains flavonol glycosides and quercetin, kaempferol and their glucosides. It also contains alkaloids:

The *Sedum* genus may contain pyrrolidine, piperidine, morpholine, indole, pyridine, thio-alkaloid and other classes of alkaloids. One sulfur-containing alkaloid 2-(2-hydroxyphenyl) benzothiazole was identified by Ligaa in 1996. Some thio-alkaloids suppress the immune system, prevent cancers metastasising, are anti-inflammatory and anti-cancer according to Matsuda in 2001.

Research

In 2016 Biagi presented a paper on *Sedum telephium's* traditional use and the pharmacological research that had been carried out on it, at the 111th Congress of the Italian Botanical Society International Plant Science Conference (IPSC,) Rome 21–23 September 2016. He treated human keratinocytes (a type of skin cell) with 0.1% *Sedum* juice for twenty four hours. He found that the *Sedum* juice stimulated the cells to synthesise almost seventy percent more collagen. Collagen is like glue, holding the cells together, so essential for wound healing. He also treated mononuclear cells (immune cells) with the *Sedum* juice and found that it stimulated the release of cytokines (immune signalling cells.)

On the 1st December 2002 The Italian company, MAG SRL Societá, patented a healing composition based on *Sedum telephium* and allantoin.

In 2010 Huang demonstrated the anti tumour activity of the Sedum genus *in vitro*. In 2008 Qin demonstrated that extracts of *Sedum sarmontosum* suppressed immune activity in mice. In 2003 Silva-Torres demonstrated the spermicidal effect of *Sedum praealtum* in mice.

How to Use Orpine

Harvest the leaves in July and August, wash and dry them and keep them in an airtight container in the freezer. Today, preparations such as a gel and a dry extract are available. Use the leaves, gel or extract to treat wounds, ulcers, whitlows, abscesses, dermatitis, burns and also to draw out foreign bodies (splinters etc.) that are embedded in the skin.

Chapter 18

Rhubarb
Rheum rhabarbarum

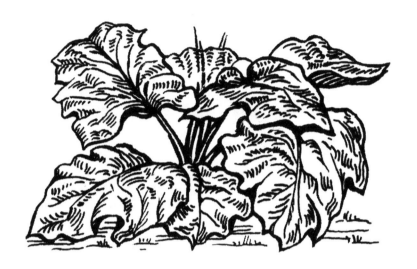

Botanical Description

Rhubarb is a collective name of various perennial plants of the genus *Rheum* L. from the Polygonaceae family. *Rheum rhabarbarum* produces large clumps of enormous leaves, up to 60cm across and proportionately huge red stems, 25mm or more in diameter and up to 60cm long, which grow from an underground stem. The leaves appear early in the spring. Later in the season a large central flower stalk may appear and bear numerous small greenish white flowers and angular winged fruits containing one seed. The roots withstand cold well, although the tops die back in autumn.

Healing Properties

Rhubarb has been used in China to treat kidney damage due to diabetes, chronic kidney failure, acute inflammation of the pancreas, gastrointestinal bleeding and other diseases, according to Jiao in 2000. In 2012 Wang described how rhubarb is used in Traditional Chinese Medicine to treat chronic kidney disease.

Rhubarb is good for digestive complaints including constipation, heartburn, stomach pain, and, surprisingly, for diarrhoea. It is a good source of dietary fibre, which can keep your digestive tract running smoothly. It staves off bloating and cramping. Some people have reported feeling less discomfort from indigestion after eating rhubarb. It can stimulate gastric juices that induce normal muscle contraction to make the digestive tract function optimally.

Rhubarb is rich in vitamin K, for brain health. Since vitamin K is associated with optimum bone density and rhubarb also contains plenty of calcium it is good for bones. The antioxidants in rhubarb are anti-bacterial, anti-inflammatory, have anti-cancer properties and help protect you from heart disease, cancer, and diabetes. They also help prevent cell damage and ward away fine lines and wrinkles that make the skin look older. Rhubarb's high vitamin A content can keep skin appearing younger longer. Rhubarb is anti-fungal and anti-viral so many folk practitioners use it to treat or prevent skin infections.

Traditional practitioners of folk medicine have long used rhubarb for its anti-inflammation benefits, whether the inflammation is caused by infection or by indigestion.

Scientists are interested in the potential anti-cancer effect of rhubarb and suggest that it could be used in new cancer treatments and therapies.

Chemical Constituents

Rhubarb contains alcohols, aldehydes, esters, keytones, acids. It contains 10–30% tannins and more than thirty anthraquinones including: rhein, emodin, aloe-emodin, chrysophanol, physcion, iso-emodin, chrysaron, laccaic acid D. Rhubarb also contains anthrones, stilbenes, polysaccharides. It is rich in antioxidants, particularly anthocyanins (which give it its red colour) and pro-anthocyanidins. These antioxidants have anti-bacterial, anti-inflammatory, and anti-cancer properties.

Research

Rhubarb is one of the most popular traditional Chinese herbs for treating damage to the kidneys due to diabetes and chronic kidney failure, according to Zhu in 2005. It is often used together with other drugs to treat diabetic kidney damage in China. In 2016 Liu found kidney function improved after treatment with rhubarb compound. In 2012 Xiong found that rhubarb reduced the excretion of urinary protein, lowered blood lipid and improved kidney function of patients suffering from diabetic kidney disease. It inhibited kidney inflammation and fibrosis.

Rhein, a component of rhubarb anthraquinones, may be responsible for protecting the kidneys. In 2004 Tan demonstrated that it protected kidney cells *in vitro*. In 2011 Su demonstrated that it inhibited the formation of kidney fibrosis in rats. In 2012 Wang found that rhein improved diabetic kidney damage in rats. In 2009 Liu found that rhein improved lipid disorders in rats. Scientists are currently studying rhein as a drug candidate to treat cancer.

Emodin, another component of rhubarb anthraquinones, has a wide range of pharmacological effects. In 2016 Cui demonstrated its anti-tumour effect in human liver cancer cells *in vitro*. In 2016 Li found that it was anti-bacterial *in vitro*. *R. rhabarbarum* is weakly anti-bacterial according to Kosikowska in 2010. In 2015 Brkanac found that it killed white blood cells and caused DNA damage at 150 micrograms per ml. In 2016 Chen demonstrated that it inhibited inflammation in rats. In 2011 Ji found that it could bring high blood pressure down and improve microcirculation.

Components of rhubarb anthraquinones: chrysophanol, physcion and aloe-emodin are anti-inflammatory. In 2016 Zhao demonstrated that chrysophanol protected the nervous system of mice against inflammation. In 2015 Tong demonstrated that physcion inhibited inflammation and protected nerves *in vivo*. In 2015 Chen found that it stopped cancer cells from reproducing. In 2015 Tabolacci found that aloe-emodin had anticancer and immunomodulatory effect on human melanoma cells.

Rhubarb contains anthrones and dianthrone which are purgative. These include rheinosides, paladin, rheidin and sennosidin. It also contains stilbenes which are antioxidant and protect the liver according to Li in 2005.

Rhubarb contains a lot of tannin. In 2006 Zhong demonstrated that this tannin was responsible for the anti-diarhoeal effect. In 2013 Zeng found that rhubarb tannins protected the kidneys of injured rats.

In 2012 Sui demonstrated that rhubarb improves blood viscosity and blood flow. In 2007 Wang demonstrated that rhubarb charcoal stopped peptic ulcer in mice from bleeding by increasing the number of platelets and reducing blood clotting time.

In 2015 Wang found that rhubarb prevented the build up of fats in the blood of rats fed a high fat diet. In 2008 Wang found that rhein and emodin prevented high blood fats and atherosclerosis in diabetic rats.

R. rhabarbarum contains natural antioxidants which act as free radical scavengers, according to Kalpana in 2012. Six stilbenes, including resveratrol are antioxidant. Seven *R rhabarbarum* compounds: i.e. piceatannol, resveratrol, rhapontigenin, desoxyrhapontigenin, pterostilbene, (E)-3,5,4'-trimethoxystilbene and *trans*-stilbene, protected the liver *in vitro* according to Dong in 2015.

Rhubarb is used to treat acute oedema and hemorrhagic necrotizing pancreatitis in China, according to Zhou in 2016. It can stimulate pancreas juice flow. In 2016 Zhou added rhubarb to somatostatin to treat acute pancreatitis. In 2017 Sun found that applying rhubarb and mirabilite externally reduced the risk of swollen abdomen, stomachache and complications in patients with acute pancreatitis. The average hospital stay was significantly shorter.

In 2013 Zhang demonstrated *in vivo* that rhubarb inhibited inflammation, improved microcirculation in the intestines and restored normal intestinal absorption. In 2015 Wang found that free rhubarb anthraquinone and rhubarb decoction could prevent kidney injury caused by acute pancreatitis.

Rhubarb is used to treat gastrointestinal bleeding clinically in China. In 2015 Wang found that conventional treatment combined with rhubarb powder was more effective at stopping upper gastrointestinal bleeding, compared with the control group in a small clinical trial.

In 2015 Wang described how rhubarb was used to treat acute organophosphorus pesticide poisoning. In 2014 Lu described using rhubarb root and rhizome to treat acute ischemic stroke.

How to Use Rhubarb

Stew or bake the rhubarb stems to release healing polyphenolic antioxidant compounds. Use rhubarb to alleviate constipation, to promote a healthy intestine and to protect the kidneys. The polysaccharides in it lower blood sugar, protect the liver, build up the walls of the intestine and protect against cancer and ageing. Of course, if you add sugar while cooking it, the blood sugar lowering effects will be cancelled.

Contraindications

You should not use rhubarb long-term since it will start to produce toxic side effects.

Chapter 19

Rose
Rosa spp

Flower of perfection, symbol of love, famed in many mythologies, highly prized by poets, the rose was dedicated to the Goddess of love and war: Ishtar in Babylonia, Isis in Egypt, Aphrodite in Greece and Venus in Rome. Ancient Muslim tradition says that the rose comes from the sweat and tears of the prophet Mohammed. As Aphrodite, the goddess of love emerged from the sea, roses grew from the foam. When she ran to save her lover, Adonis, from a wild boar sent by jealous Ares to kill him, she became entangled in thorn bushes in her haste and roses grew from her spilt blood. Dante designed paradise, in his *Divine Comedy*, in the shape of a rose.

Flowers in paintings and poetry had deep symbolic significance in Renaissance Florence. The rosebush with its "white rose of virginity, and red rose of martyrdom, the rose incarnate, born of study and of the true doctrine," as the Dominican friar Giovanni Dominici of Florence wrote, was an important element in the medieval Church iconography. Many early Renaissance paintings, such as the Madonna and Child by Domenico Veneziano, include red and white roses which represented the purity of the Virgin (the white rose) and the maternity of the Virgin (the red rose).

Alternatively the red rose could be coupled with the white lily, which represented the immaculate conception, virginity, chastity and innocence. The rose and the lily were symbolic of the Virgin Mary, who was both chaste and maternal. Padre Giovanni Pozzi (Locarno, 1923-Lugano 2002) Capuchin monk, literary critic and Italo-Swiss academic, wrote about the symbolism of flowers in his

La Parola Dipinta (the Painted Word) in 1981. He had always been fascinated by the mystic rose and conducted a flowery analysis of a Renaissance still life painting attributed to the Spanish painter Juan Fernandez el Labrador, of lilies and roses around a vase of roses. Flowers, and especially the rose, had religious, mystical and curative significance and were so important that the Duomo in Florence is called Santa Maria del Fiore and Florence itself was known as Citta del Fiore (city of flowers.)

Cosimo and many other alchemists of the time distilled rose petals for their exquisite essential oil, which would have been added to unguents, salves and lotions. Roses are mentioned seven times (always red roses) in the *spezeria* books in Florence, but the word *rosato* (containing roses or made out of roses), occurs eighty-five times. Renaissance pharmacists made rose water, rose oil, essential oil of roses, all of which were added to numerous other recipes.

Healing Properties

Rose petals lift the spirits with their perfume. They are mildly astringent and antioxidant, so can be used to strengthen a weak stomach and for diarrhoea, for sore mouth and throat. Rose hips are a valuable source of vitamin C in the winter. They are astringent, antibacterial, anti-inflammatory, antioxidant and used for colds, diabetes, diarrhoea, oedema, fever, gastritis, gout, rheumatism, sciatica. Rose hip powder, taken regularly will cure rheumatoid arthritis, prevent atherosclerosis and lessen the pain of osteoarthritis.

Chemical Constituents

Rose petals contain small amounts (0.017–0.35%) of volatile oils. These volatile oils are complex, containing at least ninety five different compounds including: citronellol, nerol, geraniol, linalool. They also contain 2.85% anthocyanins; flavonoids including: rutin, quercitrin, myricetin, kaempferol.

Rose hips contain the anti-inflammatory galactolipid: (2S)-1,2-di-O-[(9Z,12Z,15Z)-octadeca-9,12,15-trienoyl-3-O- beta-D-galactopyranosyl glycerol (GOPO), vitamin C, A, B3, D, E, phenolic compounds, and carotenoids such as: lycopene, lutein, zeaxanthin; amino acids, flavonoids, pectins, sugars, tannins, tocopherol, beta sitosterol and long-chain polyunsaturated fatty acids, magnesium and copper. The flavonoids and organic acids keep the vitamin C stable by inhibiting oxidation.

One hundred grams of Hyben Vital rose hip powder from Denmark contains five hundred milligrams of vitamin C, 5.8g pectin, 5.8mg beta-crotene, 50mg beta-sitosterol, 0.2mg folic acid, 4.6mg vitamin E, 170mg magnesium, 1mg zinc and 10.9 microgram copper.

Research
Scientists have carried out masses of research on rose hip powder, mostly looking at its anti-rheumatic properties, since it contains powerful anti-inflammatory compounds. For a full description of this research have a look at my book: *Healing Plants of the Celtic Druids*.

How to Use Rose
Collect the petals in early summer and spread them out to dry. Store in a glass container away from sunlight. Pick the hips in late autumn, early winter, when they are soft and ripe. Dry them in a warm, airy place away from the sun.

Use a tincture of roses for sore mouth and throat and as a calming digestive astringent.

Pick rose hips and make them into jams, jellies and syrups. Dry them to use in teas and infusions.

Drink rose hip tea daily to benefit your skin, since rose hips contain plenty of vitamin A, which helps to regenerate skin cells, to heal wounds and scars and to keep the skin elastic and nourished. This will not only prevent wrinkles, but can actually help to minimise any that have already appeared.

Take rose hip powder or capsules to help prevent colds and coughs and help the immune system to fight off infections. Take rose hip as a daily supplement to keep your blood vessels clear from plaque, prevent rheumatoid arthritis, ease the pain of osteoarthritis and prevent the joints from degenerating further.

Add rose essential oil to massage oil for its calming, soothing effect.

Dosage

Tincture of roses 1:1 distilled and macerated as a cordial 5–10ml per week.

Syrup of roses 30–100ml.

Rose hips infusion: 100g fresh or 45g dry.

Rose hip powder 5–10g per day.

Contraindications

Rose hips are safe if taken in moderate doses. There have been cases of people who took forty grams a day of rose hip powder, who suffered some gastrointestinal disturbances. But this is way above the recommended dose.

Chapter 20

Sage
Salvia officinalis

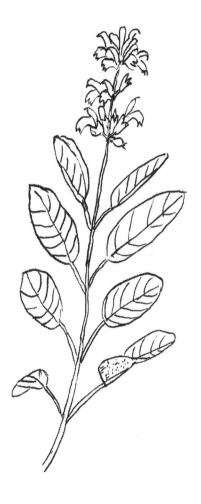

In Renaissance Florence sage was treated with religious, spiritual respect. Its Italian common name, *Salvia*, also the name of the first half of the Latin binomial, derives from the verb *salvare:* to save, mirroring the role of Jesus, the Saviour. Sometimes it was called by an alternative name: *Salvia salvatrix:* the sage of the Saviour. The species name: *officinalis* relates to its place in the *officina* of a monastery, where herbs and medicines were stored.

People associated it with wisdom and old age, partly because it could cure so many illnesses and partly because they believed that it would strengthen the brains of those who consumed it. So it was used as an ingredient in elixirs to prolong life. People also believed that sage would ward off evil and dispel ungodly spirits. No-one to date has seen fit to carry out clinical trials on sage's influence on immortality, but it does appear to enhance mental alertness and could possibly help prevent some of the ailments that occur in old age.

In Roman times those who harvested sage went barefoot, wore white robes and used bronze or silver tools in sacred ceremonies. By the Renaissance country people wearing normal clothes brought sage in to the *Oficina,* probably gathered from their gardens.

Salvia is one of the widest-spread members of the Labiatae family and there are hundreds of different *Salvia* species, which people in many countries have been using traditionally for centuries to treat a multitude of different symptoms. Most of these species have medicinal properties.

Healing Properties

Traditionally, people used sage to increase fertility, stop bleeding, heal minor skin wounds, treat hoarseness or cough, and improve memory. It is antioxidant, anti-inflammatory and sedative. It is a wonderful woman's herb, helping to regulate female hormones, especially during the menopause.

Chemical Constituents

Scientists all over the world have investigated the chemical constituents of sage. Many species of sage contain compounds that have healing properties. *Salvia officinalis* is a rich source of polyphenols; more than a hundred and sixty have been identified. Caffeic acid is the central building block of the polyphenols in sage. Two caffeic acids together form rosmarinic acid which is highly antioxidant. Three and four caffeic acids form trimers and tetramers such as salvianolic acids and lithospermic acid, which are powerful free radical scavengers. Sage contains phenolic acids such as ursolic acid, which is anti-inflammatory and salvin which is antibacterial against *Staphylococcus aureus,* the cause of upper-respiratory tract infections. It contains phenolic glucosides and glycosides of neolignans and flavonoids, such as the oestrogenic luteolin-7-O-glucoside. Most of the flavonoids are flavones of apigenin and luteolin or flavonols such as kaempferol and quercetin. It also contains methyl ethers and their glycosides, of flavones, in the leaves or in the exudate from aerial parts. It contains quercetin glycosides and their methyl ethers. *Salvia officinalis* contains condensed tannins. It also contains essential oil, composed of at least sixty eight different compounds, which is anti-bacterial. The main components are thujone, viriflorol, manool, caryophylene and humulene. It contains the cyclic monoterpenes, 1,8-cineol, pinene and camphor, which inhibit acetylcholinesterase.

Research

A great many scientists have investigated the antioxidant, anti-inflammatory and sedative effects of sage. Numerous scientists have demonstrated that sage reduces fats in the bloodstream. There has been a great deal of interest in the beneficial effect of sage on Alzheimer's disease, since sage is used traditionally to aid memory. So scientists investigated which of its chemical constituents might be responsible for aiding failing memory. They found that cyclic monoterpenes 1,8-cineole and alpha-pinene, as well as camphor, inhibited cholinesterase while 1,8-cineole, alpha- and beta-pinene were antioxidant. Since

Alzheimer's Disease (AD) is caused, in part, by compounds which oxidise and damage brain cells and since cholinesterase inhibitors are a standard treatment for AD patients, it is possible that sage might help people with Alzheimer's. But there would need to be clinical trials with sage to see whether it might be an appropriate treatment for AD patients. There has been a lot of interest in the oestrogenic effects of sage, especially on dysmenorrhoea and menopausal symptoms. For a full description of all this research see my book: *Healing Plants of the Celtic Druids*.

How to Use Sage

Take three large sage leaves and steep in boiled water for five minutes. Use this to treat indigestion, inflammation of the mouth and throat, menopausal hot flashes with excessive sweating. Add lemon juice and honey to sage leaf infusion for an effective cough mixture. Add sage leaves to food. In 1985, the German Commission E approved the use of sage internally for upset stomach or indigestion, excessive perspiration, and for sore nose and throat. The German Standard License for sage leaf infusion states that it can be used for sore gum, mouth and throat, for pressure spots caused by prostheses, and to help treat gastrointestinal catarrh (inflammation of the mucous membranes). Use sage leaf (dry extract, herbal tea, liquid extract and tincture) for:

a) symptomatic treatment of mild dyspeptic complaints such as heartburn and bloating;

b) relief of excessive sweating;

c) the symptomatic treatment of inflammations in the mouth and throat; and

d) relief of minor skin inflammations.

Chapter 21

Strawberry Tree
Arbutus unedo

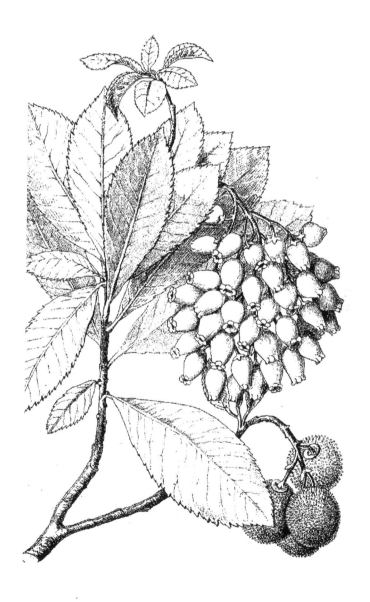

There were frequent plagues in Renaissance Florence: in 1430, 1437–38, 1449–50, 1478–79 and 1527–31. During the last period, which was during Cosimo I de Medici's reign, 20–25% of the population of Florence died. People believed that all kinds of plants would cure the plague, including the leaves of the strawberry tree. Unfortunately they were wrong.

Botanical Description

Arbutus andrachne the Greek Strawberry tree, can grow up to about 12m. The smooth bark exfoliates during the summer, leaving a pistachio green layer, which changes to a beautiful orange brown. White bell shaped flowers (resembling hot-air balloons) 0.4–0.6cm diameter in panicles of 10–30, are produced in clusters of 15–30 flowers on red stems, and are nectar-scented. The leaves are dark green and glossy, 5–10cm long and 2–3cm broad with serrated edges. The edible fruit is a spectacular red berry 1–2cm diameter, with a rough surface, which matures in 12 months, at the same time as the next flowering. Natural populations of *Arbutus unedo* are in danger due to deforestation, over-collecting and new construction on the coasts.

Healing Properties

The leaves, bark and root are astringent, antibiotic, anti-fungal and diuretic. Since they are antiseptic they are used to treat cystitis and urethritis. Their astringent action makes them useful for treating diarrhoea and, like many other astringent plants, they make a good gargle for treating sore throats. Strawberry tree fruit has antioxidant and anti-cancer properties and strawberry tree honey is a rich source of healing compounds.

Chemical Constituents

Arbutus berries contain plenty of vitamin C, malic and citric acid, as well as the minerals: potassium, calcium, phosphorus, magnesium and sodium. They are high in antioxidant phenolics, including polyphenolic flavonoids, such as +catechin, −epicatechin and arbutin. They are low in soluble sugars: fructose, glucose and sucrose. The berries have large amounts of carotenoid pigments: the major ones are (All-*E*)-Violaxanthin and 9*Z*-violaxanthin, responsible for the bright colour of the ripe fruits. In addition the berries also contain other 5,6-epoxide carotenoids, such as (all-*E*)-neoxanthin, (9'*Z*)-neoxanthin (all-*E*)-antheraxanthin and lutein 5,6-epoxide, together with lutein, zeaxanthin and β-carotene. They also contain glycosides of anthocyanins, such as cyanidin-3-galactoside. Other antioxidant compounds in this fruit were ellagic acid and its diglucoside derivative. The tree bark contains compounds such as monotropein and unidoside.

Research

Numerous researchers have demonstrated that extracts of strawberry tree leaves are antioxidant and free radical scavenging *in vitro*. This is probably due to the large amount of phenolic compounds in the extracts. Strawberry tree honey has anti-cancer effects. Several scientists have demonstrated that extracts of strawberry tree leaves are anti-bacterial. For a full account of this research see my book: *Healing Plants of Greek Myth*.

Conclusions

This is one tree that we can grow in our gardens, if we have a garden, because Strawberry trees will grow in a wide range of climates and soil types, though they do best in a nutrient-rich well-drained moisture-retentive soil in sun or semi-shade. Especially when young, they prefer a fairly sheltered position and dislikes cold drying winds. This is a very good tree to grow in towns because it tolerates industrial pollution. The white blossom and red fruit ripen in the winter and are delightfully decorative before you harvest the fruit to eat or make into jam.

Although there have not been many clinical trials to demonstrate the healing properties of the tree, people have been eating the fruit for centuries and it is perfectly safe. They have also been using the leaves, bark and root but there is insufficient evidence that these are safe.

Chapter 22

Sorrel
Rumex acetosa

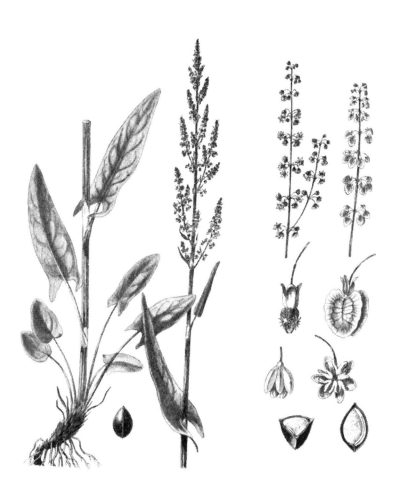

Botanical Description

Rumex acetosa is an erect perennial plant with edible, sour-tasting oblong leaves arrow-shaped at the base. The upper ones have no stalks. The flowers are in narrow panicles or racemes and as they increase in size they become a purplish colour.

Healing Properties

Sorrel is antimicrobial, antioxidant and is used for reducing sudden and ongoing pain, swelling and inflammation of the nasal passages and respiratory tract, for treating bacterial infections along with conventional medicines, and for increasing urine flow (as a diuretic). It is used to treat stomach discomfort and gastrointestinal disorders and gum disease.

Chemical Constituents

The root contains polyphenols and anthraquinones, the leaves contain dimeric and trimeric proanthocyanidins, tannins and phenolic compounds including resveratrol, vanillic acid, sinapic acid and catechin. Phenolic acids include gallic acid, protocatechuic acid, ferrulic acid, p-coumaric acid. The leaves also contain calcium, magnesium, iron, potassium, sodium, vitamin A and C and all the essential amino acids, flavonoids, such as rutin, hyperoside, quercetin, quercitrin, avicularin, vitexin, orientin and iso-orientin, which are antioxidant and anti-inflammatory.

Research

In 2001 Alzoreky found that extracts of *Rumex acetosa* were anti-oxidant. In 2012 Bae demonstrated that an extract of the plant was anti-oxidant *in vivo* and was a powerful free radical scavenger. In 2011 Gescher demonstrated that an extract *Rumex acetosa,* rich in polyphenols, was antiviral.

Gum Disease or inflammation of the gums is a very common condition and traditional healers use *Rumex acetosa* leaves to treat it. The bacterium *Porphyromonas gingivalis* is one of the main causes. Two proteinases make the bacterium stick to the cells of the gums, then invade them and modulate the local immune response. In 2013 Beckert demonstrated that a proanthocyanidin-rich extract was highly effective at inhibiting the proteinases *in vitro*. The active compounds were dimeric and trimeric proanthocyanidins. In 2015 Schmuch found that a proanthocyanidin-enriched extract of *R. acetosa* stopped *Porphyromonas gingivalis* bacterium sticking to gum tissue, again *in vitro*.

In 2012 Bae found that *R. acetosa* extracts reduced the incidence of gastric ulcers in the mice. He concluded that anthraquinones may be responsible for this. In 2016 Mimica-Dukic discovered that *R acetosa* roots were anti-inflammatory. The compounds responsible for this were the anthraquinones: chrysofanol, emodin and epigallocatechine.

Clinical Studies

Sinupret, (Bionorica SE, Neumarkt, Germany) is the brand name of an extract of Sorrel (*Rumex acetosa*), Elder flower (*Sambuci flos*), Gentian root (*Gentianae radix*), Primula flower (*Primulae flos*) and Verbena herb (*Verbenae herba*). This was formulated for the treatment of sinusitis. In 2012 Jund reported that after the extract had been evaluated *in vitro* and *in vivo* and found to be anti-inflammatory, anti-viral and anti-bacterial, it was tested in clinical trials, which demonstrated that 160mg taken three times for fifteen days was an effective cure for acute viral rhino-sinusitis.

How to Use Sorrel

Add a few sorrel leaves to salads.

Take sorrel tablets, such as Sinupret (Bionorica SE; Neumarkt, Germany), a proprietary blend of botanicals, for sinusitis and bronchitis. Tablets contain 18–36mg of sorrel leaf and stem extract, in addition to four other herbs: elder flower (*Sambucus nigra*), primrose flower and calyx (*Primula veris*), European vervain leaf and stem (*Verbena officinalis*, Verbenaceae), and yellow gentian root (*Gentianalutea*). Do not take the tablets long term.

Contraindications

In 1998 Brinker reported that if you eat a large amount of sorrel (*Rumex acetosa* L.) this may lead to dermatitis, diarrhoea, gastrointestinal problems, polyuria and nausea. He also says that when taking pharmaceutical drugs together with *R. acetosa* there may be precipitation of these drugs due to high tannin content of sorrel. It contains oxalic acid (300mg per 100g of sorrel), which can precipitate calcium in human blood leading to serious kidney damage. If you suffer from kidney stones avoid sorrel. Eating herbs such as sorrel over long periods can cause damage to the absorption of calcium and iron in the human body. Cooking it decreases the concentration of oxalic acid.

Both domestic poultry, goats and sheep have been poisoned by eating too much sorrel because of its high level of oxalic acid.

Part 3

Exotic Healing Plants Used in
Renaissance Florence

Cosimo I de' Medici sought out every exotic plant he could
find, growing whatever he could in his gardens.

Chapter 1

Balm of Gilead
Commiphora gileadensis

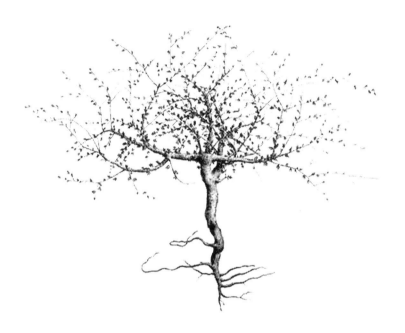

Balm of Gilead, or balm of Mecca, is the resin from *Commiphora gileadensis* of the Arabian Peninsula. Ancient writers, such as Josephus Flavius, Pliny the elder, Pedanius and Gaius Tacitus, highly praised the balm (balsam) tree of Judea, as a holy oil, a cure for many diseases, and as a perfume, according to Zohary in 1982. Dioscorides said the balsam had the most powerful healing properties, followed by the seeds, then the wood. When the balsam tree bark is cut the sap flows out as an oil. It is fresh, strongly fragrant, liquid, a little astringent and soluble in water. If left in the air it soon hardens with a sweet smell and quickly evaporates. The hardened resinous gum tastes like lemon or pine resin when chewed. People also burn it as incense. It was produced in Ein-Gedi and Jericho during the Second Temple, Roman and Byzantine eras, according to Hepper in 2004. People also use the shoots in folk medicine to treat various illnesses according to Lev in 2002. Traditional Arabic medicine uses the flower and leaf decoctions as an analgesic and to increase bowel movement and diuresis according to Abdul-Ghani in 1997. In Saudi Arabia today *Commiphora gileadensis* is considered an important medicinal plant, according to Al-seini in 2014 and used to treat swelling, pain and fever, according to Al-Howiriny in 2004. Modern scientists are generally ignorant of the history and elaborate folk medicinal value of this species.

Botanical Description

Commiphora gileadensis, also known as *Commiphora opobalsamum,* is a member of the resinous plant family Burseraceae, comprising, among others, the Biblical frankincense and myrrh. It is native to southwest Arabia and Somaliland, where it grows as a thornless bush 1.5m high, or small tree 5m high, under arid tropical conditions. It has a reddish or grayish bark. Its white flowers grow in small clusters and produce ovoid or ellipsoid, smooth, glabrous fruits which contain a fragrant yellow seed that brightens in colour as the seed matures and dries.

Healing Properties

Commiphora gileadensis is wound healing, anti-inflammatory, anti-fungal and anti-bacterial. It will also heal ulcers if taken internally and will relieve muscle and joint pain.

Chemical Constituents

Commiphora gileadensis contains flavonoids, tannins, steroids, amino acids, triterpene glycosides, saponins and a volatile oil in which myrcene is the major compound, plus beta and alpha pinene, alpha phellandrene, simonene, copaene, elemene, allo-ocimene, alpha-thujene, sabinene and n-nonane. It also contains several semi-volatile sesquiterpenes; alpha-gurjunene, beta-ylangene, trans-beta-caryophyllene, allo-aromadendrene, and delta-cadinene; monoterpenes and alkanes.

Research

In 2022 Alhazmi found that *Commiphora gileadensis* speeded up wound healing, was anti-inflammatory and antibacterial in mice. In 2010 Gilboa-Garber demonstrated that it was anti-bacterial *in vitro*. In 2015 Al Mahbashi found that it was antibacterial against a range of bacteria, most strongly against *Staphylococcus aureus*. It was also anti-fungal against *Candida spp.*

In 2005 al Howiriny found that pre-treating rats with balsam extract protected them from ulcers.

In 1997 Abdul-Ghani found that *Commiphora gileadensis* extracts were anti-inflammatory and protected the liver of rats. He found that extracts of the leaves and flowers brought down blood pressure of rats. In 2016 Anwar also found that *C gileadensis* protected the livers of rats. He suggested this was due to the antioxidants in the plant such as flavonoids, volatile oils, saponins, triterpenes and sterols, since they work as free radical scavengers. He also demonstrated that the plant was safe.

Healthy skin involves a balance between creating new skin cells which rise to the skin surface, where they divide into different types before dying and flaking off. Inflammatory skin diseases such as psoriasis are associated with an imbalance between these processes and skin cancer cells manage to avoid programmed cell death. In 2010 Chan found that the best way to kill cancerous cells is to do it while they are dividing, when they are at their most vulnerable. So with this in mind, in 2015 Wineman collected growing tips from a *Commiphora gileadensis* plant, cut them and collected the sap, diluted it in ethanol and made an extract. Thinking that the extract might be selectively toxic towards cells that were dividing, he compared its effect on skin cancer cells and normal human skin cells. He found that it killed 65% of the skin cancer cells but left the normal skin cells unharmed.

In 2008 Shen isolated several new triterpenoids, sesquiterpenoids and glycosides from *Commiphora gileadensis*. He found that these compounds destroyed human prostate, liver and cervical cancer cells. β-caryophylleneone is the key cancer cell killing component. Many spice blends citrus flavours, soaps, detergents, creams, and lotions, as well as in a variety of food and beverage products contain β-Caryophyllene, which is also anti-inflammatory, local anaesthetic, and anti-fungal.

In 2020 Haddad demonstrated the anti-diabetic effect of *C gileadensis* in rats.

Unfortunately there have been no clinical trials to demonstrate the wound-healing and anti-ulcer effect of *C gileadensis*.

How to Use Balm of Gilead

Use Balm of Gilead oil to massage painful arthritic joints. It will relieve inflammation and reduce pain. It soothes skin irritations such as eczema, cuts, rashes, burns, psoriasis, insect bites and stings, sunburn, athlete's foot, dry and scaly skin, chapped hands or cheeks, and heals diaper rash. Apply the oil or ground up resin to wounds to prevent infection and speed healing.

Contraindications

Do not take internally.

Chapter 2

Camphor Tree
Cinnamomum camphora

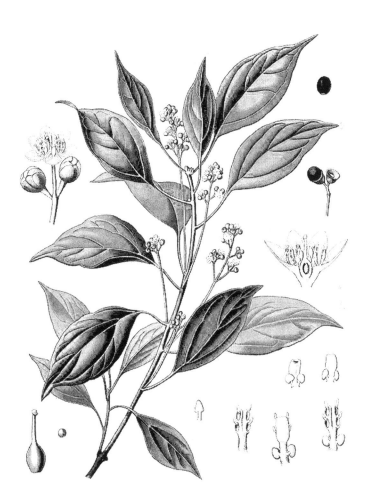

There are about 200–350 species of the genus *Cinnamomum*, widely distributed in South East Asia. Camphor trees (*Cinnamomum camphora*) are native to China, India, Mongolia, Japan and Taiwan and grow in the tropical rain forests at various altitudes from highland slopes to lowland forests including marshy places and on well-drained soils. People now cultivate *Cinnamomum camphora* in China, Taiwan, southern parts of Japan, Korea, and Vietnam. They have been distilling the wood, twigs and bark for centuries, to obtain camphor, a white, crystalline substance with a strong smell and pungent taste. People have been using it throughout the world to treat a variety of symptoms such as inflammation, indigestion, infection, congestion, pain, irritation, etc., according to Zuccarini in 2009.

The camphor tree or camphor laurel, *Cinnamomum camphora* is one of the tree species that were intentionally introduced to Australia in the nineteenth century to enrich the flora of the Australian colonies. It flourished, especially in wet, coastal eastern Australia, where it now dominates the landscape in many places, and has come to be considered an environmental weed.

Botanical Description

The camphor tree is broad-leaved and evergreen and grows up to 20m, with a stout, uniformly cylindrical bole and dense, symmetrical crown. It is handsome, shapely, resilient and every part of it smells of camphor. It has pale brown bark, entire leaves 4–10cm, whose upper sides are glossy dark green, duller green underneath, which grow alternately, sometimes with wavy margins. The flowers are small, greenish white and grow in panicles, followed by 1cm small purple berries with a single seed.

Healing Properties

Camphor is antispasmodic, stops itching, is anti-inflammatory, contraceptive, antiseptic, mild expectorant, nasal decongestant, will suppress a cough and prevent infection. It will absorb through the skin, so can be rubbed on as a topical analgesic, according to Sydney in 1978.

Chemical Constituents

There are several varieties of camphor (*Cinnamomum camphora*) with different chemical constituents, according to Frizzo in 2000. The main constituent of *Cinnamomum camphora* leaf is camphor, together with cineol, linalool, eugenol, limonene, safrole, alpha-pinene, beta-pinene, beta-myrecene, alpha-humulene, cymene, nerolidol, borneol, camphene and some other components.

Research

There has been a great deal of research into the healing properties of camphor, almost all of it carried out in the laboratory, on cell cultures and unfortunate rodents. I'm not going to attempt to cover it all. In 1990 Ghanta found that when he exposed mice with cancer to vaporised camphor it delayed the growth of the cancer. In 1998 Elizabeth Kaegi developed a drug called 714-X based on camphor which some institutions believe is effective against breast and prostate cancer. In 2011 Padma demonstrated that Padma 28, another multi-herbal remedy containing camphor, was effective against inflammatory diseases in diabetic mice. In 2012 Salman showed that camphor leaves protected mice from DNA damage caused by Atrazine, a common herbicide. In 1996 Ling demonstrated that two proteins from camphor: cinnamomin and camphorin, inhibited carcinoma cells. They also demonstrated that cinnamomin stopped solid melanoma from growing in mice. In 2002 Liu stated that cinnamomin and camphorin, two ribosome-inactivating proteins, are storage proteins in camphor tree seeds. These compounds are toxic against viruses, tumour cells, insects and plant fungi.

Carbon nanotubes are being developed for the medical profession, to deliver drugs more efficiently. Normally these nanotubes are synthesised from petroleum products, but in 2003 Kumar demonstrated that camphor could be used to create them. This would be an environmentally-friendly alternative starting material. Camphor is a cheap botanical hydrocarbon which is already cultivated, according to Kumar in 2007. He suggested that cultivation could increase.

Camphor essential oil contains monoterpenes, which inhibit human cancer cells such as: colon cancer, gastric cancer, liver tumour, breast cancer, leukaemia and other cell lines, according to Edris in 2007. Most cancer chemotherapy is highly toxic to both the cancer cells and healthy cells, which has a terrible effect on the body. Scientists have tentatively suggested that camphor essential oil containing monoterpenes could suppress tumours without causing so much harm.

The camphor tree is a member of the Lauraceae, a plant family that often has anti-oxidant, anti-inflammation and anti-tumour effects, according to Lin in 2007. In 2009 Chen-Lung and team distilled the essential oils from the leaves, flowers and twigs of *Cinnamomum camphora* and tested them for anti-oxidant and anti-fungal effects. They were able to isolate and identify several compounds, including linalool and camphor in the flowers and twigs. The twig essential oil was the most anti-oxidant, whereas the leaf essential oil was the most powerfully anti-fungal.

In 1995 Ansari demonstrated that camphor oil repelled mosquitoes. Since several species of mosquito transmit dangerous diseases, such as malaria and Dengue fever, mosquito-repellent oils are important, especially ones that can replace the harmful synthetic agents currently in use.

2009 Zuccarini demonstrated that treating patients with camphor before giving them radiation reduced the growth of the cancer.

In 1993 Burrow asked a group of people suffering from colds and blocked noses to inhale camphor vapours for five minutes to see whether it would help to clear their noses. He found that it had no effect on nasal resistance to airflow but the majority of the people reported that their noses felt cooler and they felt they could breathe better. Burrow concluded that camphor stimulates the cold receptors in the nose.

Proper clinical trials are needed to demonstrate how effective camphor could be for the treatment of several conditions.

How to Use Camphor

Put two or three pieces crystalline camphor in your tea light candle diffuser and let the candle vaporise it to purify the air and bring peace and tranquility to the environment. Use the vaporised camphor to ease the congestion of a cold. Dilute camphor essential oil in a carrier oil: 20% camphor oil to 80% carrier oil and massage the joints to relieve pain of osteoarthritis, fibrositis, neuralgia and the itching of insect bites. It will increase blood flow to the skin and act as a counterirritant. Massage onto the chest to relieve chest congestion, cough, bronchitis and asthma. Be very careful not to exceed the dose of camphor essential oil in the carrier oil because camphor is toxic in large doses. Several over-the-counter products contain camphor and should be used with care.

Contraindications

Avoid camphor during pregnancy, because it crosses the placental barrier. Do not give it to children who are prone to febrile convulsions. Do not eat camphor. Cases of camphor intoxication in humans, especially children, are relatively frequent, mostly because people have accidentally eaten it. Avoid synthetic camphor, which is highly toxic. Natural camphor occurs as D-camphor. Camphor can be synthesised in the laboratory, but only as L-camphor, which is far more toxic than D-camphor. Be careful always to source your natural camphor from a reputable provider.

Chapter 3

Cinnamon
Cinnamomum verum

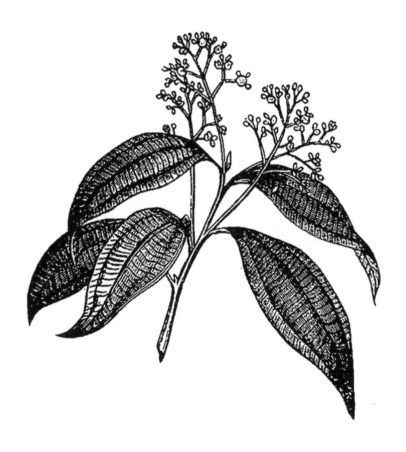

Growing up on a farm in Kent, our parents took us carol singing in December, driving through the snow in the Land Rover, up to a farmhouse, where we sang our carols in four part harmony, breathing in the icy air on the blackest of nights. Lights would come on and the farmer's wife would invite us all in to offer us mince pies and mulled wine, heavy with the scent of cinnamon and clove and sweetened with honey. Back in the Land Rover we continued on our way to the next farmhouse and more mulled wine.

Good quality cinnamon, *Cinnamomum verum*, the third most important spice in the world, is native to Sri Lanka, while poorer quality cinnamon from other *Cinnamomum spp* is called cassia. People use whole *Cinnamomum verum* bark in food and drinks. An essential oil and an oleoresin are used as medicine. Ancient Egyptians used cinnamon as an embalming agent; it was brought to Europe from Asia as a cooking spice and medicine.

Botanical Description

Cinnamon trees grow 10–15m high with thick scabrous bark, strong branches, young shoots speckled green orange, with ovate to oblong leathery leaves, whose upper side is shiny green and underside is lighter. The flowers are small white and grow in loose, branching clusters. The fruit is an oval berry with a receptacle like an acorn, bluish when ripe with white spots on it, bigger than a blackberry. The root-bark smells like cinnamon and tastes like camphor, which it yields when distilled. When you bruise the leaves they smell spicy with a hot taste. Commercial cinnamon bark is the dried inner bark of the shoots.

Healing Properties

The German Commission E approved the internal use of both *C verum* and *C aromaticum* to treat loss of appetite, dyspeptic complaints such as mild spastic conditions of the gastrointestinal tract, bloating, and flatulence. Cinnamon is powerfully antioxidant, anti-inflammatory, anti-bacterial and lowers cholesterol. It modulates the immune system and kills mosquito larva. Some compounds in cinnamon have anti tumour action. Eating cinnamon makes you feel full sooner and keeps the food in the stomach longer, prevents the oxidation of fats, enhances insulin signalling and glucose transport, alters carbohydrate metabolism and glucose absorption. Traditional healers use it to alleviate arthritis, high blood pressure, dermatitis, toothache, colds, for improving menstrual irregularities and for wound healing.

Chemical Constituents

Cinnamon bark consists of a variety of resinous compounds, including cinnamaldehyde, the main constituent and cinnamate, cinnamic acid, and 1–2% essential oils which contain: eugenol, L-borneol, caryophyllene oxide, b-caryophyllene, L-bornyl acetate, e-nerolidol, α-cubebene, α-terpineol, terpinolene, and α-thujene, trans-cinnamaldehyde, cinnamyl acetate; also coumarin, tannins, cinncassiols, melatonin, procyanidins and catechins.

Research

Spices such as cinnamon contain antioxidants and when used in food they protect our health. They protect us from free radicals which damage our cells and tissues, causing metabolic diseases and age-related syndromes. One of the things antioxidants do is to prevent fats from being oxidised, which is why they are sometimes added to fats and oils. This is important because oxidised fats stick to the walls of the blood vessels, causing atherosclerosis. In 2000 Shobaba found that cinnamon extracts prevented fats from being oxidised. Several scientists, including Mancini-Filho in 1998, have demonstrated that *Cinnamomum zeylanicum* is antioxidant. In 2001 Okawa found that flavonoids isolated from cinnamon were antioxidant. He demonstrated *in vitro* that they scavenged free radicals. In 2002 Lee isolated trans-cinnamaldehyde from *Cinnamomum cassia* bark and found that it was powerfully antioxidant.

Several scientists, including Tung in 2008, demonstrated that the essential oil of *Cinnamomum osmophloeum* was anti-inflammatory *in vitro*. Lin in 1999 demonstrated that cinnamon is anti-inflammatory due to the flavonoids in it which are also antioxidant.

In 1994 Yu isolated cinnamophilin from *Cinnamomum philippinense* and demonstrated that it protected rat brains from damage due to lack of oxygen. In 2009 Lee found that cinnamophilin reduced brain damage in rats caused by starving the brain of oxygen and glucose.

Two percent of people over the age of sixty-five suffer from Parkinson's disease, the second most common nerve-degenerative disease after Alzheimer's. In 2009 Brahmachari found that sodium benzoate, a compound from cinnamon, reduced inflammation in brain cells *in vitro*.

Sixty to eighty percent of dementia cases are caused by Alzheimer's disease. It is caused (at least in part) by beta-amyloid plaques accumulating in the brain. In 2011 Frydman-Marom demonstrated that cinnamon extract reduced these plaques from forming in the brains of mice and improved cognitive performance.

In 2013 Hossein found that distilled cinnamon speeded up blood clotting time *in vitro*. In 2001 Chang found that essential oils of *Cinnamomum osmophloeum* were antibacterial *in vitro*. In 2005 Wang demonstrated *in vitro* that *Cinnamomum osmophloeum* essential oil was anti-fungal.

In 2006 Kim demonstrated that cinnamon extract had an anti-diabetic effect in mice. In 2005 Park demonstrated that *Cinnamomum verum* oils killed nematodes *in vitro*. In 2004 Cheng found that essential oils from *Cinnamomum osmophloeum leaves* killed mosquito larvae. In 2009 Lu demonstrated the anticancer effect of cinnamon extract.

In 2012 Hwa demonstrated that a compound from *Cinnamomum cassia* protected rat hearts from damage caused by heart attack. In 2013 Song found that two compounds, cinnamic aldehyde and cinnamic acid, isolated from *C. cassia* protected rat hearts from myocardial ischemia (lack of oxygen to the heart). They proposed that cinnamon could be used to treat cardiovascular diseases. Several studies have reported that cinnamaldehyde protects the cardiovascular system. In 1975 Harada found that cinnamaldehyde from Chinese cinnamon also protected the cardiovascular system.

In animal studies, cinnamon decreased smooth muscle contractions in the trachea and ileum, colon, and stomach.

In 2014 Mansoure gave cinnamon and lemon balm tea to 32 glass production workers in the morning and evening for thirty days. After treatment, the high-density lipoprotein (good fats) and antioxidants significantly increased in their blood. The workers' ability to think and perform tasks improved. Since cinnamon and lemon balm contain plenty of antioxidants he suggested that this tea could be used to protect workers from oxidative stresses.

In 2010 Abascal cited a review of studies investigating a formula including cinnamon which reduced the symptoms of angina.

Women suffering from dysmenorrhea experience painful cramping, nausea and heavy menstrual bleeding. In 2019 Singletary reviewed the five small clinical trials using cinnamon to treat this condition. Scientists gave patients cinnamon doses from 999–1500mg/day for periods of 2–6 months. 3 of the trials showed improvements in insulin sensitivity, compared with controls. In 2 of 3 trials, the women who took the cinnamon had lower levels of fasting blood glucose, and lower levels of low-density lipoprotein (bad fats) compared with controls. In another study women taking cinnamon to treat dysmenorrhea noticed less pain and nausea. One woman suffered a rash and itchiness but none of the others noticed any side effects. In another recent review, scientists included cinnamon in many of the formulas used to treat of endometriosis.

However, none of these studies used enough women, and none lasted more than four months. All the studies used different species of cinnamon, which, although they contain mainly the same compounds, do not contain the same amounts of each compound. Plant portion, quality of grade, species/varieties of cinnamon, and processing and extraction of cinnamon powder all have an impact on the chemical composition of the sample used in the trial. Few of the studies reported the chemical composition of the samples the participants took. This information would be helpful in providing information about the active compounds. To truly evaluate cinnamon as a treatment for dysmenorrhea larger studies need to be carried out, with a specific species of cinnamon whose chemical composition has been identified, and for longer periods, in order to identify any possible side effects.

Good quality cinnamon bark, *Cinnamon verum* is generally regarded as safe. *Cassia cinnamon,* however, should be avoided, due to its high coumarin content.

How to Use Cinnamon

Use good, *Cinnamon verum* in cooking. It is best to buy the bark and grind it in a coffee grinder or a pestle and mortar since you can never be sure that the cinnamon powder you buy is true cinnamon and not inferior cassia. Also ground cinnamon loses much of its potent aroma over time, so it is best to use it freshly ground. Use the whole bark steeped in hot drinks, such as mulled wine or apple juice where it will impart its wonderful flavour. Add it to food and it will keep the food in your stomach longer and make you feel full sooner and protect your blood vessels from harmful oxidised fats.

Make an infusion of cinnamon bark to treat mild spastic conditions of the gastrointestinal tract, loss of appetite, bloating and flatulence.

Dosage

Dried herb: 0.5–2g 3 times a day.

Essential oil: 1 to 3 drops 3 times a day.

Make an infusion with 5g in a cup of boiled water and take 3 times a day.

Tincture (usually 1:5, 60%–80% ethanol with some glycerine added to prevent precipitation of tannins): 1–3ml 3 times a day.

Contraindications

Cinnamon contains coumarin. *Cassia cinnamon*, a common ingredient in foods in the US, contains a great deal more coumarin than Ceylon cinnamon *Cinnamomum verum*. Consuming too much coumarin can lead to liver damage and affect the ability of the blood to coagulate.

People should speak to their doctor before adding cinnamon or cassia to their diet if they take anticoagulants or other drugs, have diabetes or a liver condition.

Chapter 4

Dragon's Blood Tree
Dracaena draco

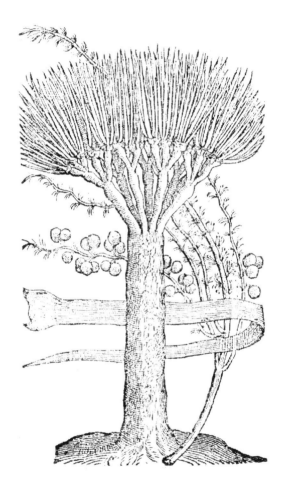

I encountered the Canary Islands dragon tree when I spent the winter in La Palma, living in a cave and working for the wonderful Frohmut and her outdoor cafe, overlooking the steep barrancos leading to the sea below. The dragon trees were unlike anything I had ever seen, like giant mushrooms stretching up into the sky, their blood-red trunks below thick green canopies of leaves, often clinging to the narrowest of ledges on the steep hillsides.

In Renaissance Florence people used dragon's blood: a translucent, film-forming resin with a natural red colour from the Canary Islands' dragon tree. They used it in medicine, in lacquers, as an artist's colour and for ritual magic. Alchemists described its origin as the combined blood of dragons and elephants fighting to the death.

Doctors and herbalists revered dragon's blood for its magical restorative properties and believed it was a universal remedy. It is not unlikely that the artists who used the resin thought it endowed their work with special, magical properties, for the colour red symbolised the red elixir in the final stage of the alchemical work, when the divine tincture could restore man to perfect health and consciousness of God. One alchemical image is of a dragon and a rooster being eaten by a fox which is being eaten by another rooster. The dragon represents dragon's blood. The sun indicates gold. The fox represents acids dissolving gold and the rooster eating the fox shows a circular process. Gold is dissolved and re-dissolved by nitric and hydrochloric acids, chlorine builds up and the gold volatilises into gold chloride, which is red.

There are sixty to a hundred different *Dracaena* species, of which only six are trees. These include *Dracaena cinnabari,* which grows on the Socotra island off the coast of Yemen and *Dracaena draco,* native to the Canary Islands, Madeira and Cabo Verde.

Botanical Description

Dragon trees belong to one of the oldest ecosystems in the world and have survived the glaciations of the Oligocene to Miocene and are now endangered. They are monocotyledons: plants whose seeds only contain one embryonic leaf or cotyledon, as opposed to dicotyledons, which have two cotyledons in their seeds. Almost all trees are dicotyledons with rings which mark their growth. The dragon tree has no growth rings and we can only estimate its age by counting the number of its branches. It belongs to the Agave family.

Dracaena draco can grow up to twenty metres high and has aerial roots which sometimes merge with its trunk. Its scaly bark is reminiscent of a dragon. The densely packed green crown of the tree is shaped like an open umbrella. These trees grow slowly from the top of the trunk, branching to produce the umbrella-shaped crown, and can live up to six hundred years. In the first ten to fifteen years only the trunk grows, then it begins to form branches. The branches also grow for ten to fifteen years, before splitting again. It takes a century for the crown to reach its beautiful umbrella shape. The leaves at the end of the branches grow in dense rosettes and are shed every three or four years before new leaves simultaneously mature. The leaves are stiff, 30–60cm long and 2–3cm wide. The fragrant, white or green flowers grow in groups of 2–3 at the end of the branches.

Healing Properties

Dragon's blood, the sap from the tree, will stop bleeding, is anti-diarrhoea, anti-ulcer, anti-bacterial, anti-viral, wound healing, anti-tumour, anti-inflammatory and antioxidant.

Chemical Constituents

The resin is rich in flavans, homo-iso-flavans and -flavones, chalcones and dihydro-chalcones, including unique compounds called dragonins, sterols and terpenoids

Research

In 2015 Shu described how a patient suffering from bed sores was treated with dragon's blood applied externally, combined with conventional treatments, such as oxygen, vacuum aspiration and anti-infection therapies. The patient made a complete recovery from the bed sores. In 2011 Gupta found that Dragon's blood resin from *Dracaena cinnabari* was antioxidant and antibacterial. In 2016 Ansari demonstrated that extracts of *Dracaena cinnabari* resin from Soquotra Island, were effective against multi-drug-resistant bacteria. In 2011 Silva demonstrated that *Dracaena draco* fruit was antioxidant.

Very little research has been done on the medicinal properties of the Canary Island dragon tree: *Dracaena draco,* although people have been using its resin since ancient times as a traditional medicine to stop blood flowing from wounds, to cure diarrhoea, to treat ulcers and as an antibiotic, antiviral, wound healing, anti-inflammatory, antioxidant, according to several authors, including Gupta in 2008 and Milburn in 1984. Several scientists, including Gupta in 2008, demonstrated that steroidal saponins extracted from *D draco* stopped myeloid leukaemia cells from growing and increasing. In 2003 Gonzalez isolated two steroidal saponins called draconins A and B from *D draco* bark which killed leukaemia cells. Several scientists, including Camarda in 2011, have isolated flavans, methylflavans, flavanones, homoisoflavans, homoisoflavones, chalcones, dihydrochalcones and other compounds from *D draco* resin. In 2007 Melo identified dracoflavylium, the major red colourant. In 2014 Di Stefano collected resin from *D draco* trees growing in the Botanical Garden of Palermo and isolated sixteen known flavones and chromones from the resin. He demonstrated that extracts of the resin were antibacterial.

Conclusions

Since so little research has been carried out into the safety and efficacy of dragon's blood, I cannot advise anyone to take it internally. And since the dragon trees are endangered, perhaps we should not be using their resin at all.

Chapter 5

Lemon Grass
Cymbopogon citratus

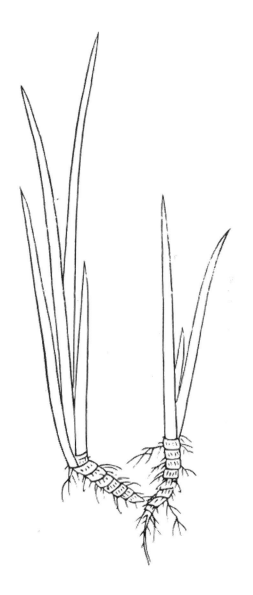

In Vietnam, Laos and Cambodia we used to eat delicious food, flavoured with lemongrass, sometimes wrapped in a banana leaf to keep all the lovely flavours in. I had no idea, at the time that it was so medicinal. Years later, in Sri Lanka I remember going to the local shops to buy little bottles of citronella oil (the essential oil of lemongrass) that we all rubbed on our exposed skin in the evenings to deter mosquitoes. I thought it smelled wonderful, though not everyone agreed with me, but it was effective.

The name *Cymbopogon* comes from the Greek word *kymbepogon*, which means boat-beard. It may also be referred to as ginger grass or citronella grass. It is a perennial fragrant grass, that people now cultivate throughout tropical America and Asia. In the Philippines people cook the heart and young shoots as a vegetable.

This would have been one of the plants that Cosimo I's gardeners grew in terracotta pots and brought indoors in the winter, for it doesn't survive frost.

Botanical Description
Lemongrass belongs to the Gramineae family and is probably native to South India, Malaysia and Sri Lanka. It is a tropical, evergreen, perennial, aromatic grass that can reach up to 1.8m and will continue to grow for several years in dense clumps. It has several stiff stems and slender, blue-green, blade-like leaves which droop towards the tips. The leaves turn red in autumn and smell strongly of lemon when damaged. It produces large compound flowers on spikes.

Healing Properties
Lemongrass is antioxidant, anti-amoebic, anti-bacterial, anti-diarrhoeal, anti-filarial, anti-fungal and anti-inflammatory. Traditional healers in south east Asia use the leaves and the essential oil to relieve spasms, increase perspiration and to treat

indigestion, arthritis pains, and various skin conditions. The perfumery industry uses the essential oil in perfumes, cosmetics and soaps. Lemon grass is used in traps to attract swarms of insects.

Chemical Constituents

Lemongrass contains terpenes, including limonene, ocimene, alpha pinene, alpha caryophylene, phellandrene, oxobisabolene; triterpenoids, such as cimbopogone; alcohols, ketones, such as methylheptenone; and esters. The essential oil consists mainly of citral. Active compounds include myrcene, which is antibacterial and pain reliever; citronellal, citronellol, geraniol and citral and an aldehyde with strong lemon fragrance..

Research

Scientists have carried out a great deal of research into the medicinal properties of lemongrass extracts, essential oil and isolated compounds, in the laboratory.

In 2006 Tangpu demonstrated that lemongrass extract and citral were anti-diarrhoeal in mice. In 2010 Figueirinha demonstrated *in vitro* that lemongrass leaf infusion was anti-inflammatory. In 2000 Viana demonstrated that lemongrass essential oil was anti-nociceptive in mice (it stopped them feeling pain.)

In 1976 Seth demonstrated that lemon grass essential oil depressed the central nervous system of mice and Ferreira found that it prolonged sleep time for mice. The tea, however, did not have the same sedative effect, according to Carlini in 1986. In 1990 Rao found that myrcene prevented mice from feeling pain. In 2000 Viana found the same thing. They noticed that the analgesic effect did not cause tolerance to develop when they repeated the doses, unlike morphine. However, Moron Rodrigues in 1996 found that fluid extract of lemon grass did not have an analgesic effect in rats.

Several scientists have looked at the anti-cancer effect of lemongrass extract, including Kauderer in 1991 who found that alpha myrcene was anti-mutagenic in mammary cells. In 1993 Zheng found that limonene and geraniol, isolated from lemongrass, inhibited liver and intestinal cancer cells. In 1994 Vinitketkumnuen found that lemongrass extract was anti-mutagenic *in vitro*. In 1994 Murakami registered that lemongrass had some anti-tumour properties. In 1997 Suaeyun demonstrated that lemongrass extract inhibited colon cancer in mice. Also in 1997 Dubey found that citral, isolated from lemongrass, killed leukaemia cells *in vitro*.

A great many scientists, including Danlami in 2011, have demonstrated that lemongrass extracts were antibacterial. In 2012 Silva found that lemongrass oil and citral were anti-fungal against *Candida spp in vitro*. Scientists have known for a long time that essential oils containing a lot of citral are anti-bacterial and anti-fungal. Guenther wrote about this in his book on essential oils in 1950. In 1984 Onawunmi isolated geranial and neral from lemongrass, demonstrated that they were also anti-bacterial and that myrcene reinforced this effect when added to the other compounds. In 1992 Ibrahim tested lemongrass essential oil against 20 bacteria, 7 yeasts and 15 fungi and found that the bacteria were more susceptible than the fungi. Several scientists, including Baratta in 1998, have demonstrated that lemongrass oil was anti-bacterial and antioxidant. Several scientists, including Syed in 1995, have demonstrated that lemongrass essential oil was anti-fungal.

A number of scientists, including Ansari in 1995, have demonstrated that lemongrass essential oil repels mosquitoes, while Tchoumbougnang in 2005 demonstrated that lemongrass essential oil was anti-malarial in mice. Onabanjo in 1993, on the other hand, found that aqueous extract of lemongrass was antimalarial in mice.

Several scientists, including Baratta in 1998 have demonstrated that lemongrass essential oil was anti-oxidant.

How to Use Lemon Grass

Make an infusion of the dried leaves and drink warm when you have a cold, since it will help reduce mucus. It is good for stress, so take when you have a headache. It will help the digestive system and ease abdominal cramps, colitis, indigestion, gastroenteritis and rheumatic conditions. It will help to digest fats and cut down cholesterol levels, rid the body of toxins and promote heart health.

Add a few drops of the essential oil to a carrier oil and massage to relieve tension and stress.

Rub the essential oil onto your exposed skin to keep mosquitoes away, especially when you are in tropical countries, to avoid catching dengue fever and malaria.

Use the fresh leaves in cooking, if you can find them.

Chapter 6

Lignum vitae
Guaiacum officinale

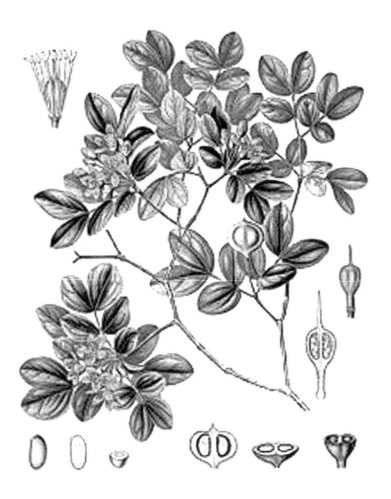

Lignum vitae is wood from the Tree of Life, or *Guaiacum officinale*, a wood so dense that it sinks to the bottom when you put it in water, a wood so resistant to rot, that posts for dwellings in Tutu, St Thomas were carbon dated to 800 years old. The tree is native to the Caribbean, southern Florida, the west coast of Central America and the north coast of South America. The genus, *Guaiacum*, comes from the tree's Caribbean name. It is the national flower of Jamaica.

Guaiacum is a native Bahaman word, adopted in Europe in the sixteenth century and the word guaiac refers to resin from trees of the Genus *Guaiacum*. There are five species of *Guaiacum*, two of which: *Guaiacum officinale* and *Guaiacum sanctum* were imported to Europe from the Dominican Republic in 1508 between the rule of Lorenzo the Magnificent and Cosimo I de' Medici. They renamed the wood *lignum sanctum* (holy wood), *lignum vitae* (wood of life) and *lignum indium* (Indian wood), although the trees did not come from India. It was used to treat syphilis, also newly arrived in Europe from Latin America.

Christopher Columbus's crew picked up syphilis on the island of Hispaniola (Haiti and the Dominican Republic) and brought it back to Spain in 1493. When the French army invaded Italy some Spaniards in the French army infected prostitutes in Naples. From there it spread like wildfire throughout Italy and the rest of Europe.

Lignum vitae, which was used to treat syphilis in central and south America, soon acquired a reputation as a cure for it. Since it was a new disease, few people fully understood it. Nicholas Pol, a physician, sent a report to Cardinal Lang who was investigating the healing properties of guaiacum for syphilis, on June 22, 1516, with a recipe for guaiac treatment that he acquired from a spice dealer from Seville.

In 1519 Ulrich von Hutten published *De guaiaci medicina et morbo Gallico* in which he talked about his own case of syphilis and how he cured himself with guaiacum. He boiled shavings of the holy wood in water to make a thick black liquid which he drank regularly for forty days in a heated room where he stayed immobile. This, he said, was what the natives of the Caribbean did to cure the disease. His paper was reprinted in many languages, and doctors all over Europe began to treat their syphilitic patients with strong enemas and sweating in hot, dark rooms for forty days, after a strict fast, according to Eppenberger in 2018. They fed guaiacum potions to their patients and rubbed guaiacum ointments on the affected parts. So many people contracted syphilis that demand for guaiacum grew immensely and twenty-one tons of it were imported to Spain between 1568 and 1608.

Many famous people, such as Cesare Borgia, according to Sarah Dunant in 2013, Ivan the Terrible, Prince of Moscow (1530–1584), King Henry III and Charles V of France, Maria Salviati (1499–1543), wife of Giovanni de' Medici of the Black Bands, Isabella of Aragon (1470–1524) and Maria of Aragon (1503–1568) according to Antonio Fornaciari in 2020. All the noblewomen were infected by their husbands.

Johannes Stradanus (1523–1605), whose patron was Francesco de Medici, made a collection of engravings known as *Nova Reperta* (New Discoveries). The sixth engraving is called *Hyacum et lues venerea* (*Guaiacum and venereal disease*). One half of the picture depicts a man cutting wood chips from a guaiacum log, a woman weighing it and another woman boiling it up. The other half of the picture shows the sick man in bed drinking the decoction while the physician stands over him and an attendant stands ready to refill his cup. There is another painting of an amorous encounter, which explains how the man became ill.

The reason why people thought that guaiacum cured the disease was because they did not understand that the symptoms naturally occur in three episodes, between which they disappear. At the time the only other treatment was mercury, which caused horrendous side effects. This made guaiacum seem like an attractive alternative.

Paracelsus, born Theophrastus von Hohenheim (1493–1541), a voice crying in the wilderness who had understood the nature of the disease, tried to publish the truth: that the guaiacum treatment for syphilis was a scam. But the Fuggers family, who were making shedloads of money through their monopoly of the guaiacum trade, succeeded in convincing the Leipzig Faculty of Medicine to prohibit publication of Theophrastus's paper. Not only were the Fuggers importing the Holy Wood and selling it at hugely inflated prices, they had also set up a hospital called the *Blätternhäuser* (pox house) or the *Holzhaus* (woodhouse) where patients suffering from syphilis were treated with guaiacum at huge expense.

By the eighteenth century people had realised that guaiacum did not work against syphilis, so imports came to a halt, according to Gaenger in 2015. In 1864 Isaac Van Deen discovered that guaiacum could be used to detect blood in the urine and faeces, since the haem in haemoglobin from the blood oxidises guaiac acid to guaiac blue. All of a sudden people were interested in guaiacum again.

Botanical Description

Guaiacum officinale is a slow growing evergreen tree, eventually reaching about 10m with a greenish-brown trunk with a diameter of 60cm. The leaves are compound, 2.5–3cm long and 2cm wide. The attractive flowers, with five bluish purple petals, fading to white are about 2.5cm across. The fruit is bright yellow-orange with red flesh and black seeds.

Healing Properties

Guaiacum wood and resin possesses anti-cancer, anti-bacterial, anti-oxidant and anti-cholesterol properties. People make medicinal extracts from the wood and resin for muscle and rheumatic joint pain, breathing problems and skin disorders.

Chemical Constituents

In 2004 Ahmad isolated a number of saponins, including a new triterpenoid saponin: guaianin from *Guaiacum officinale* bark.

The bark also contains alpha and beta sitosterol, oleanic acid, a saponin, officigenin and furoguaiaoxidin, a new enedione lignan.

Research

In 2017 Maneechai extracted the bark, twig and leaves of *Guaiacum officinale* L. (Zygophyllaceae). He found that the extracts were anti-oxidant and free-radical scavenging. In 2021 Shoukat identified anti-cancer, anti-bacterial and anti-oxidant principles in *Guaiacum officinale* fruits. In 1994 Duwiejua demonstrated that *Guaiacum officinale* was anti-inflammatory in rats. In 2003 Offia and Ezenwaka described how they gave extract of leaves, flowers, fruits and twigs of *Guaiacum officinale* to pregnant mice and rats. It caused abortion in many of the rodents and significantly reduced the litter size. They suggested that these findings supported the traditional use of *Guaiacum officinale* as an anti-fertility drug. I'm not sure whether they meant that people used guaiacum to abort unwanted pregnancies, or to prevent conception occurring in the first place. In 2014 Lowe found that leaf, seed and twig extracts of *G officinale* inhibited HIV1. In 2014 Bahada-Sing demonstrated the wound healing properties of *Guaiacum officinale* in diabetic rats. In 2018 Ibrahim demonstrated that *Guaiacum officinale* extract protected the pancreas of rats from diabetes induced damage.

Contraindications

I would not advise taking guaiac wood or resin internally or using products based on this plant externally. All the research has been carried out in the laboratory either *in vitro* or on unfortunate rodents and although it appears to have some anti-cancer possibilities it is clearly toxic. During the Renaissance people believed that it could cure syphilis, which was why it was included in the plants used by the Medici.

Chapter 7

Liquorice
Glycyrrhiza glabra

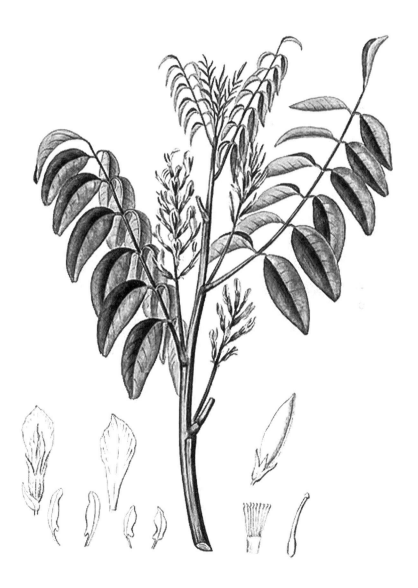

There are about twenty species of *Glycyrrhiza*, belonging to the legume family (Fabaceae.) The most famous member of the genus is *Glycyrrhiza glabra*, liquorice, a perennial herb native to the Mediterranean region, central to southern Russia, and Asia Minor to Iran.

People have been using liquorice in China since 3000 BCE and the Chinese Pharmacopeia states that it soothes irritation and is added to cough mixtures, either as a tincture or fluid extract. Dioscorides named the plant *Glyrrhiza:* Greek *glukos*, sweet, and *riza*, a root. Assyrian clay tablets recorded its use in 2500 BCE. According to Bruneton in 1995 people used it in ancient Arabia to treat coughs and to relieve diarrhoea caused by laxatives. Theophrastus used it to treat dry cough and asthma in 372 BCE while Pliny the Elder stated that liquorice was expectorant and carminative according to Dr Marderosian in 1999. Piero de Cresenzi of Bologna described its cultivation in Italy in the thirteenth century. It relieves spasms of the gastrointestinal tract, according to Tu in 1992. The Indian Ayurvedic Pharmacopoeia states that it is expectorant, demulcent (soothing), anti-spasm, anti-inflammatory, an adrenal agent, and a mild laxative, according to Karnick in 1994. The Indian Pharmacopoeia says it is demulcent. The extracts are still used to flavour food and liqueurs.

Botanical Description
Liquorice plants are graceful, with light, spreading, pinnate foliage, looking almost feathery from a distance. The leaflets (like those of the False Acacia) hang down during the night on each side of the midrib, not quite meeting underneath it. Racemes or spikes of papilionaceous small pale-blue, violet, yellowish-white or purplish flowers grow from the axils of the leaves. The seeds develop in small pods similar to partly-grown pea-pods. The species *glabra* has smooth pods, hence the

specific name. Other species of *Glycyrrhiza* have hairy or spiny seed pods.

Liquorice roots grow both downwards as tap roots, and horizontally as rhizomes or stolons, for many metres. These runners have leaf-buds and sprout up as stems in their second year. Both the downward tap roots and the long, horizontal stolons are used medicinally.

Chemical Constituents

The roots and stolons contain about 59% by weight, glycyrrhizin, a saponin about 50 times sweeter than sucrose. Glycyrrhizic or glycyrrhizinic acid is the main metabolite of glycyrrhizin. Flavonoids include: liquiritin, isoliquertin, liquiritigenin and rhamnoliquirilin, glucoliquiritin apioside. Flavonones include prenyllicoflavone A, shinflavanone and rhamnoglucoside, liquiritigenin. Isoflavans include glabrene. Coumarins include licopyranocoumarin, licoarylcoumarin, glisoflavone and new coumarin- GU-12. They also contain a chalcone, lipochalcone A. semilicoisoflavone B, 1- methoxyficifolinol, isoangustone A, and licoriphenone, as well as volatile oil, which contains: pentanol, hexanol, linalool oxide A and B, tetramethyl pyrazine, terpinen-4-ol, α- terpineol, geraniol and others.

Healing Properties

Liquorice is anti-inflammatory and used to treat arthritis. It is expectorant, soothing, controls coughing, is used to treat bronchitis and is often an ingredient of cough mixtures. It detoxifies and protects the liver. People use it to treat Addison's disease and asthma. Liquorice has a mild laxative effect and can protect the lining of the gut by increasing the production of mucus, thus alleviating heartburn and ulcers. It has hormonal effects and is also used to treat allergic complaints.

Research

Scientists have carried out masses of research into the healing properties of liquorice, especially in China and Japan where it has been used medicinally for many centuries. It contains several active compounds according to Kaur in 2013: the flavonoid, glabridin has anti-ulcer effect, may enhance memory and is active against mycobacteria, the bacteria that cause tuberculosis; licochalcone A is anti-malarial; the flavonoid, liquiritin is anti-spasmodic; the flavonone, rhamnoglucoside is a muscle relaxant; the isoflavan, glabrene and the flavanone liquiritigenin are oestrogenic. Its most important compounds are glycyrrhizin and its main active metabolite, glycyrrhetic acid, which protect the liver, are anti-inflammatory, anti-cancer, anti-viral, anti-thrombin, anti-HIV, anti-hepatitis C, lower blood glucose, suppress coughs and stimulate the immune system.

Hepatitis C virus can lead to chronic liver disease which in turn can cause liver cancer, one of the most common cancers in the world. Glycyrrhetic acid is similar in structure to adrenal gland hormones. It inhibits the liver's metabolism of aldosterone, so effectively acting as though it were stimulating aldosterone. Since it inhibits hepatitis C virus, doctors in Japan give glycyrrhizin to patients with the virus. They report that it reduces the chances that the virus progresses to liver cancer. So in 1999 Van Rossum carried out a double blind clinical trial with fifty seven hepatitis C patients divided into four groups. He gave them either 240, 160 or 80mg of glycyrrhizin or placebo three times a week for four weeks. During treatment Hepatitis C decreased in the groups taking the glycyrrhizin.

In Japan they have developed a new drug from glycyrrhizin called Stronger Neo-Minophagen C (SNMC) which they now use to treat hepatitis C. In 1997 Arase gave SNMC to 453 patients with chronic hepatitis C, daily for eight weeks, then two to seven times a week for 2–16 years. Another group of 109 patients (Group B) could not be treated with SNMC or interferon for approximately nine years and were given other herbal medicine (such as vitamin K). After ten years 7% of the SNMC group had developed liver cancer while 12% of the other group had developed liver cancer.

In 1993 Acharya gave SNMC to eighteen patients with subacute liver failure due to viral hepatitis for 30 days. 72% of the patients survived, compared with only 31% of patients in an earlier trial who did not receive the SNMC. In 1997 Pompei found that glycyrrhizic acid was active against several viruses, including Herpes simplex, which it completely destroyed.

In 1994 Numazaki injected SNMC into three infants whose livers were enlarged due to cytomegalovirus (CMV) infection. After the course of treatment their livers had become normal.

In 1991 Akamatsu demonstrated that glycyrrizin inhibited neutrophils (white blood cells) from generating reactive oxygen species. This means that glycyrrizin has an anti-inflammatory effect similar to hydrocortisone. Other anti-inflammatory effects of glycyrrizin include inhibition of cyclo-oxygenase and prostaglandin as well as indirectly inhibiting platelet aggregation, according to Wang in 2001.

In 1991 Nagai demonstrated that glycyrrhizin protected rats' livers from damage. This may be due to liquorice isoflavones, hispaglabridin A and B inhibiting oxidation of fats in the liver cells.

All this research indicates that Glycyrrhiza glabra is an important healing plant, used for centuries to treat many diseases. *In vitro* and animal studies have shown that both the whole root and individual compounds in it have many important therapeutic properties according to Kaur in 2013.

More and larger clinical trials need to be carried out.

How to Use Liquorice
Take liquorice root as a tea, a tincture, a powder or a supplement. Add it to cough mixtures. Take it to calm your intestine, detoxify

your liver, stimulate the walls of your intestine to increase the production of mucus, alleviate heartburn and ulcers.

World Health Organisation (WHO) and European Scientific Committee of Food recommend taking no more than 100mg per day. Do not take for prolonged periods since chronic use and large doses of the root can cause severe fluid and electrolyte imbalances.

Contraindications

Since liquorice acts like the hormone, ACTH, it causes sodium retention, potassium depletion, and water retention. Never take too much liquorice because it could cause high blood pressure and muscular weakness.

Liquorice interacts with blood thinners, cholesterol lowering medications, including statins, diuretics, oestrogen-based contraceptives and non-steroidal anti-inflammatory drugs. If you are taking any of these do not use liquorice. Children, pregnant and breastfeeding women, and those with kidney disease, heart disease, or high blood pressure should avoid liquorice products.

Chapter 8

Nutmeg
Myristica fragrans

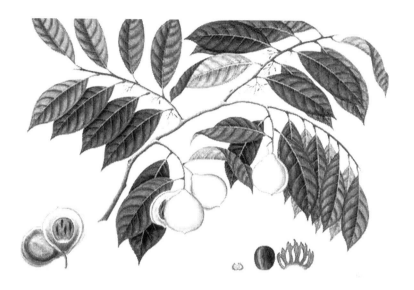

The history of nutmeg is a long, complex and bloody one, involving several European countries and a tiny group of islands in what is now Indonesia.

The nutmeg tree is a native of the Banda Islands in the Maluku Province of Indonesia, a group of ten small volcanic islands, two thousand kilometers east of Java. The Banda Islands formed part of an Asian trading network that connected Java with the Philippines and the South China Sea, and since the time of Christ, according to Ellen in 1993, these islanders, who were master navigators, traded all kinds of luxuries, such as bird of paradise feathers, nutmegs and cloves. The Bandanese soon realised the importance of the nutmeg and began cultivating it, which led to the Banda Islands becoming key ports for the nutmeg trade with Chinese, Malay and Javanese. The Bandanese, who lived in autonomous villages, each run by *Orang Kaya* (rich men), became wealthy through trade and competed with each other for power.

In 540 CE Actius of Constantinople recorded the appearance of nutmeg, according to Battaglia in 2018, who also writes that, "Arab traders [most probably] brought it to Europe from the Moluccas via Java and India." Indeed, its name, *Myristica*, could be a derivative of the Arab word *mesk*, meaning musky or fragrant.

Eventually the Europeans found the spice islands; first the Portuguese in 1511, when they conquered Malacca (now in Malaysia.) They heard that nutmeg grew on the Banda Islands and went in search of it, since it was as valuable as gold. They finally reached the islands in 1512 and spent a month filling their ships with nutmeg, mace and cloves.

Ternate and Tidore are two small Banda islands almost facing one another, each shaped by a volcano emerging from the deep Maluku Sea. These tropical paradise islands with thick forests covering the steep slopes of their volcanoes competed for trade. Their big mistake was to ask European powers to help them defeat each other. The *Orang Kaya* of Ternate invited the Portuguese to help him defeat Tidore and Tidore sought help from the Spanish. The Portuguese took advantage of the situation, creating a base in Ternate, conquering other islands and installing an *Orang Kaya* who was loyal to them. Ternate became the most powerful Moluccan sultanate. The Portuguese sent their ships laden with nutmeg, mace and cloves, all the way back to Europe, a long and dangerous journey, round the Cape of Good Hope, where many a ship was destroyed by fierce storms. Cosimo de Medici heard about this wonderful spice and acquired it for his *Spezeria*.

The Bandanese islanders put up with the Portuguese in Ternate, until they committed the heinous crime of killing the *Orang Kaya* in 1570 (and, according to several sources, cutting him to pieces and salting him in a barrel.) His son, Babullah, was so enraged that he laid siege to the fort where the Portuguese were living. Then he campaigned around the Moluccas, driving out the Portuguese and forcing Christian communities to convert to Islam. In 1575, the Portuguese surrendered the fort and were evicted from the island.

The English and the Spanish made it to the Moluccas in the 1570s and 1580s. The Dutch arrived in the 1590s and founded the Dutch East India Company in 1602. The *Orang Kaya* of Ternate asked them to help him get rid of the Portuguese and by 1605 the Dutch had replaced the Portuguese as rulers of the area. Then in 1606 the Spanish allied themselves to the sultan of Tidore and attacked Ternate, taking control of the island. The Ternatans asked the Dutch to help them defeat the Spanish but their army was too small so they built an alternative fort on the other side of the island and took control of the north, leaving the Spanish entrenched in the south. The *Orang Kaya* of Ternate signed a treaty giving the Dutch East India Company a monopoly on buying cloves and nutmegs from all the islands belonging to Ternate. The Banda islanders, however, continued to sell spices to everyone, behind the Dutch backs, while Tidore signed treaties with the Spanish, causing friction between the Dutch and Spanish for the next decades.

When a Dutch official showed up in 1609 with 1,000 soldiers and Japanese mercenaries, furious with the local *Orang Kaya* for breaking their monopoly deals, the Bandanese tricked him into leaving most of his weapons and troops on a beach and walking inland to meet them. Then they massacred this force, initiating a series of open conflicts with the Dutch.

The Portuguese, who had been ejected from the Moluccas, did not abandon the spice trade. They switched to buying spices in Makassar, in south Sulawesi. This was now an international trading port where European traders customarily bought rice to exchange for spices in the Banda Islands.

In 1613 the Dutch withdrew from Makassar and concentrated on the Moluccas. They asked the sultan of Makassar to stop trading with the Moluccas. He famously replied: 'God made the land and the sea, divided the land among the people, and gave the sea in common. It has never been heard that anyone has been prohibited from navigating the sea. If you would do it, you would take the bread out of the mouths of people. I am a poor king.'

In 1616 the Dutch sent a warning letter to the English threatening violence if they (the English) came near the Moluccas. The Banda Islanders continued to repel the Dutch and trade with whoever they liked. So in 1621 Jan Pieterszoon Coen, head of the Dutch East India Company, attacked Banda Besar, the largest island and hotbed of resistance, with one thousand six hundred Dutch troops and eighty Japanese mercenaries. The islanders resisted fiercely but were defeated within days. Coen burnt their villages and enslaved almost eight hundred people. Many Bandanese jumped off cliffs rather than surrender. By the end of this bloody war only a thousand Bandanese remained across all ten islands. There were about fifteen thousand in the year 1500.

The Company then created nutmeg plantations, imported slaves to work in them and tried to maintain a monopoly on the spice trade. Even after this brutal and openly genocidal Dutch campaign the Banda islanders did not vanish from history, but slipped to the peripheries of Dutch control to run new nutmeg trading operations.

European and Asian traders continued to trade in spices through Makassar in south Sulawesi. The Dutch East India Company tried to enforce their monopoly through violence but Makassar resisted successfully with their formidable armies.

In 1677 the Dutch traded Manhattan to the British for just one Banda Island, a barely one-square-mile speck of land. They did so because these ten obscure islands on the southeastern edge of modern Indonesia were thought to be the world's sole source of nutmeg, one of the most valuable commodities in Western Europe.

In the early nineteenth century the British conquered all the islands in the region. They transplanted nutmeg trees to Penang, Sri Lanka, Bencoolen and Singapore before handing back the islands to the Dutch in 1814. From there nutmeg trees were transplanted to Zanzibar and Grenada.

Now it is cultivated in Grenada, India, Sri Lanka, Mauritius, South Africa and the US according to Francis in 2019. The Banda islanders' regional trade dominance outlasted the colonial nutmeg craze. At least two Bandanese villages survive to this day, carrying on old traditions on the nearby Kei Islands.

It takes seven to nine years before nutmeg can be harvested from the trees and they do not reach full production for twenty years. The nutmeg seed has outer, red arils called mace and an inner, brown kernel called nutmeg, both of which are used as a spice. People dry the seeds in the sun for six to eight weeks until the nutmeg has shrunk away from its seed coat and the kernels rattle in their shells. Then they break the shells with a wooden club and remove the nutmegs. The crimson-coloured seed coat, or aril, is flattened out and dried for ten to fourteen days.

Ayurvedic doctors use nutmeg to treat anxiety, nausea, diarrhoea, cholera, stomach cramps, parasites, paralysis and rheumatism. People also use it as an aphrodisiac according to Gils and Cox in 1994. Nutmeg essential oil is used in perfumery.

People in search of a nutmeg high eat or smoke the grated spice since it contains myristicin, a natural compound with mind-altering effects, similar to LSD, if ingested in large doses. The high can last up to two days. Dr. Jeffrey Bernstein, medical director at the Florida Poison Information Center at Jackson Memorial Hospital said: "...most people only try it once because they have such nasty side effects. The rewards are not worth the risks." Bernard Sangalli, director of the Connecticut Poison

Control Centers, said that, though fairly uncommon, nutmeg abuse is periodically rediscovered.

Botanical Description

The nutmeg tree in the family Myristicaceae likes to grow in areas about one thousand three hundred metres altitude. It is an evergreen tree, fifteen metres tall, with a conical shape with a grey-brown trunk and dark green glossy leaves. The branches of the tree spread in whorls and the leaves are oval or lanceolate, glossy and grow alternately from the branches. They are dark green above and paler underneath and 10–15cm long. The leaves have petioles about 30cm long. The flowers are fragrant, and grow on short stalks of about equal length at equal distances along an elongated stalk. Male and female flowers are yellow, small and rise from the leaf base and very similar in shape and colour with minimal differences. The fruit is a round pendulous drupe, composed of a succulent pericarp. The seed is fleshy, firm, whitish, transversed by red-brown veins, rich in oil. Dried nutmegs are greyish brown, ovoid with furrowed surfaces, about 20.5–30mm long and 15–18mm wide, weighing 5–10g. Mace, the seed coat, changes colour from red to pale yellow, orange or tan and consists of flat, smooth, horn-like, brittle pieces about 40mm long.

Chemical Constituents

Nutmeg is rich in carbohydrates, proteins, dietary fibre and vitamins A, C. and E. It also contains sodium, potassium, calcium, copper, iron, magnesium, manganese, zinc, phosphorus, carotene-B and crypto-xanthin B. It has 30–40% fats, also called nutmeg butter, which contains butyrin and myristin. It has 10% essential oils which contain terpenes (α-pinene, p-cymene, sabinene, camphene, myrcene and γ-terpinene) terpene derivatives (terpinol, geraniol, and linalool) and phenylpropanes (myristicin, safrole, and elmicin.)

The essential oil of nutmeg grown in the West Indies has different proportions of the active compounds from that grown in the East Indies. There is a higher percentage of almost all the active compounds in the East Indian nutmeg. Battaglia states that nutmeg essential oil is frequently adulterated with tea tree (*Melaleuca alternifolia*) essential oil.

Healing Properties

Nutmeg is antioxidant, anti-bacterial, anti-fungal, anti-depressant, aphrodisiac, and carminative. It is also good for digestion, getting rid of gas and stomach ache, relieving vomiting and diarrhoea, as well as encouraging appetite. Nutmeg can also help with coughs and colds and is often an ingredient in cough syrups. It is a tonic for the cardiovascular system, according to Balick in 2000. It increases blood circulation and stimulates the heart. Herbalist, Chevallier in 2016 recommends using nutmeg for digestive issues, insomnia, rheumatism and eczema. Nutmeg essential oil is anti- inflammatory, anti-convulsant, antioxidant, digestive, emmenagogue, anti-emetic, anti-rheumatic, antispasmodic, a prostaglandin inhibitor, stimulant and a tonic.

In 2015 Eric Yarnell recommended using nutmeg to aid falling asleep in his article: Herbal Medicine for Insomnia. In 1932 Robert Tisserand stated in the international Journal of Aromatherapy that nutmeg oil can significantly increase happiness and calmness and decrease embarrassment and anger.

Research

Atta-ur-Rahman demonstrated that the essential oil of nutmeg was anti-fungal *in vitro*. In 2011 Gupta demonstrated that essential oil of nutmeg and several compounds in it, such as beta caryophyllene and eugenol were antioxidant *in vitro*. In 2010 Calliste stated that lignans from nutmeg are metabolised in the human body to produce antioxidant compounds. In 2008 Checker demonstrated *in vitro* that aqueous extract of nutmeg and mace protect cells from DNA damage caused by radiation. This is due to the lignans in nutmeg and mace. In 2007 Cho found that nutmeg extracts were antibacterial. Myristic acid and trimyristin were the main antibacterial compounds. They isolated three lignans from a nutmeg extract (meso-dihydroguaiaretic acid, nectandrin-B and erythro-austrobailignan-6) which were anti-fungal. In 2004 Dorman isolated carvacrol, gamma-cumene, alpha-pinene, beta-pinene and beta-caryophyllene from the essential oil of nutmeg. He found the all these compounds were antioxidant and antibacterial. In 2006 Sabulal found that anti-fungal and anti-inflammatory activity of plant essential oils were due to beta-caryophyllene. In 2000 Dorman demonstrated that the volatile oil of nutmeg was anti-bacterial against twenty-five different bacteria, including animal and plant pathogens, food poisoning and spoilage bacteria. He found that alpha-pinene and beta-pinene were strongly antibacterial. Carvacrol kills bacteria in the same way as other phenolic compounds, by destroying their cell membranes, according to Ultee in 2002. Gamma-cymene works synergistically with carvacrol, enlarging and weakening the cell membranes of bacteria. In 2007 Bounatirou proposed that antibacterial activity is due to both major and minor compounds working together.

In 1991 Hussain found that extract of mace prevented cancer in mice. In 1994 Kyriakis demonstrated that essential oil of nutmeg protected the livers of rats. Nutmeg is active against colon cancer and breast cancer, according to Malik in 2022

Inflammation plays an important role in various diseases such as rheumatoid arthritis, atherosclerosis and asthma. Several authors reported that nutmeg and its oil were anti-inflammatory, including Mueller in 2010. In 2000 Olajide demonstrated that nutmeg oil was anti-inflammatory and as analgesic and antipyretic as non-steroidal anti-inflammatory drugs in rats. It was also anti-thrombotic and anti-diarrhoeal. In 2010 Zang demonstrated that nutmeg oil could alleviate chronic inflammatory pain in rats.

In 2010 Nguyễn found that nutmeg extract activated an enzyme that could help cure type-2 diabetes and obesity. He isolated seven compounds: tetrahydrofuroguaiacin B, 2,5-bis-aryl-3,4-dimethyltetrahydrofuranlignans, fragransin C1, saucernetindiol, nectandrin B, verrucosin, galbacin and nectandrin responsible for this effect.

In 2022 Vasantrao Padol carried out a clinical trial on sixty participants suffering from plaque and plaque-related halitosis. She diluted nutmeg oil to make a mouth wash which she gave to half the participants. She gave the other half chlorhexidine gluconate mouthwash. She treated both groups for twenty-one days twice a day. She found that the nutmeg mouthwash was as effective as the chorhexidine gluconate. In 2019 Shetty carried out a trial on thirty young, periodontally healthy subjects to test the antibacterial properties of nutmeg mouthwash. First the mouthwash was tested *in vitro* against *Prevotella intermedia* (Pi), *Porphyromonas gingivalis* (Pg), and *Aggregatibacter actinomycetemcomitans* (Aa), all bacteria that can infect the mouth. The nutmeg mouthwash killed them effectively. The subjects were divided into two groups and half were given nutmeg mouthwash and the other half chlorhexidine mouthwash. Shetty found that the nutmeg mouthwash was as anti-bacterial as the chlorhexidine but less effective at preventing plaque.

In 2019 Samaranyake carried out a small randomised trial on thirty young women with acne. The patients were given a traditional face cream containing nutmeg and curd (yoghurt) which they applied to their faces at night for three months. At the end of this period their acne had improved.

How to Use Nutmeg

Safrol and eugenol, two compounds in the essential oil, are possibly carcinogenic. Therefore Tisserand and Young advise using only 0.8% East India nutmeg oil diluted in a carrier oil for massage and 5% similarly diluted for the West Indian nutmeg essential oil. These are tiny amounts. So if you are using East Indian nutmeg essential oil you'll add just under 1ml to 100ml of carrier oil. For the West Indian nutmeg you'll add 5ml to 100ml carrier oil. You can dilute the nutmeg essential oil in sunflower oil, body butter, lotions or creams. Massage aching joints and feet after exercise. Use as aromatherapy massage to lower high blood pressure, ease stress, tension, worry and depression.

Put a few drops of nutmeg essential oil and a few drops of lavender oil in your infuser to create an uplifting, soothing and relaxing ambience or to help you go to sleep.

Make an infused nutmeg oil (not to be confused with essential oil of nutmeg) by grinding two whole nutmegs in a coffee grinder, then adding the nutmeg powder to 170ml sunflower oil in a jar. You can, of course, add other herbs to the oil, such as rose petals, calendula flowers, St John's wort flowers. Store in a dark cupboard for 6–8 weeks, shaking the jar from time to time. Strain through muslin and store the resultant oil in another jar in a cool, dark, place.

To make a salve take 85g of beeswax and melt in a Bain Marie. When melted stir in 170ml nutmeg oil (not essential oil of nutmeg) and 170ml calendula oil. Pour into glass jars and cap. Store in a cool, dark place and use this salve for pain, inflammation, stomachache and stress or just for a quick-pick-me-up when life overwhelms. Apply a small amount of salve to painful places. Dab wrists and inhale for stress and anxiety release. Massage a small amount of salve clockwise over abdomen for stomach upsets.

Add ground nutmeg to coffee, tea or other warm drink. Sprinkle it on vegetables, cereals, fruit, add it to baked goods.

Always freshly grate your nutmeg, organic if possible, on your finest grater. Use in very small quantities.

Contraindications

Do not consume exaggerated amounts of nutmeg powder, since it can cause giddiness, tingling, euphoria and hallucinations, including distortion of time and space, detachment from reality, sensation of separation from one's limbs and fear of impending death. Other unpleasant side effects include headache, nausea, vomiting, abdominal pain, dizziness, chest pain, flushing, tremor, tachycardia, palpitations, agitation, anxiety, dry mouth, chest tightening and blurred vision. Ten grams (approximately two teaspoons of ground nutmeg or two whole nutmegs grated) is enough to cause some or all of these symptoms. At doses of 50 grams or more, those symptoms become more severe: alternating delirium and extreme drowsiness, eventually leading to death.

Chapter 9

Senna
Cassia angustifolia, Cassia senna (syn. Cassia acutifolia, Senna alexandrina)

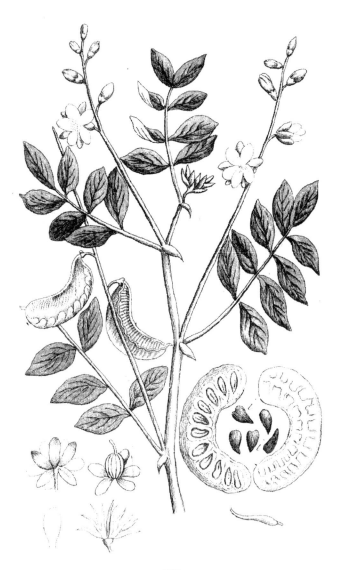

Cassia, a medicinal plant unknown to Dioscorides, was extremely popular in Renaissance Florence. It is mentioned twenty-one times in the Florentine *spezeria* since doctors at that time believed in purging practically all their patients. It appears in the account book in diverse forms, as a pulp, an oil, a preparation mixed with other herbs and so on.

The word *Cassia* is derived from the Greek *kasia* (aromatic shrub). The word senna is derived from Arabic *sanaa* (thorny bush). People in the parts of the world where it grows have been using senna as a medicine for thousands of years. In 2009 McGovern analysed residues from 3150 BCE Egyptian pottery jars and found that they had contained wine and medicinal herbs. It was difficult to discover exactly which herbs but there is a possibility that senna was one of them. The Ebers Papyrus 1550 BCE seems to describe senna, according to Aboelsoud in 2010.

Arab traders who travelled between the Roman Empire and India, transporting different species of senna, were responsible for introducing it both to India and Europe, in the eleventh century, according to Warmington in 1928. In the ninth century CE Serapion the elder of Baalbek (Lebanon) recommended using it as a medicine and Yitzhak ben Shlomo ha-Yisrael, also known as Isaac Judaeus, who also lived in the ninth century, wrote that senna from Mecca was the best quality.

Linnaeus listed twenty six *Cassia species* including *Cassia senna* in his *Species Plantarum* in 1753.

There were about 330 *Cassia* species, but plant taxonomists moved 300 of them to the genus *Senna* while 30 remain in the genus *Cassia,* according to Nesbitt in 2010. *Cassia angustifolia* from India and *Cassia senna* from Sudan, Egypt, Eastern Africa and Hejaz (a region in western Saudi Arabia) are used in Europe and America but many other types of senna are used medicinally, such as *C occidentalis* in Ghana, Senegal senna (*C italica*) in Mali, purging senna (*C fistula*) in Ayurvedic Pharmacopoeia, and so on.

Europe and the US classify it differently. In the US senna refers to *Senna alexandrina* which is confusing because *Cassia angustifolia, C acutifolia* and *C senna* are still synonyms for *Senna alexandrina*. In the European Pharmacopoeia *C angustifolia* and *C senna* are different species, with different geographic origins and contents of active principles.

Cassia senna was called Alexandrian senna because it was exported from the Egyptian port, according to Wood in 1833. It came from the southern part of the Eastern Desert, part of the Sahara between the Nile and the Red Sea. In the Sudan it was called Khartoum senna and grew in the Nubian Desert. It also grew in Eritrea, Djibouti, Somalia and Kenya.

There are three main producers and exporters of senna leaves and pods: India (cultivated only), Sudan (mostly wild harvested and some cultivated), and Egypt (wild harvested and cultivated). India is now the world's largest senna-producing region, with a cultivation area of about 22,000 hectares (54,363 acres). Since the mid-2000s, India has been increasing the cultivation of certified organic senna steadily. Before 2000, there was almost no certified organic senna in the global market.

In Sudan senna pod is a major export, along with gum arabic and hibiscus. Of course, there has been almost constant fighting in the Sudan for many years, which makes the collection of senna a difficult and dangerous occupation.

In Egypt various terrorist organisations in the areas where senna is produced make life difficult for the senna collectors, such as bedouin shepherds living in the Wadi Allaqi, a dry river in the southeastern part of the Eastern Desert of Egypt. The Egyptians are starting to cultivate organic Senna. Even in India the senna-producing area is not free of problems because it is so near the border with Pakistan, where terrorist organisations operate and where both countries' militaries are on perpetual high alert.

Botanical Description

Cassia angustifolia and *Cassia senna* are perennial under-shrubs about 1–2m high, adapted to survive with little water, with smooth, pale green trunks and long, spreading branches. The leaves are pinnate with four or five opposite paired lanceolate leaflets 20–50mm long and 7–20mm wide at the centre in the case of *C angustifolia*. *C senna* leaflets are 15–40mm long and 5–15mm wide. Dried pods of *C senna* are 40–50mm long and at least 20mm wide with six to seven seeds. *C angustifolia* pods are 35–60mm long and 14–18mm wide with five to eight seeds.

The flowers have five yellow petals, five sepals and grow in racemes at the ends of the branches with ten straight stamens. The fruit is a legume pod with several seeds.

Chemical Constituents

The primary active compounds in senna are hydroxyanthracene glycosides (HAGs.) These include dianthrone glycosides (including sennosides A, A1, B, C and D) and anthraquinone glycosides. The leaves and pods contain slightly different amounts of these compounds. Senosides A and B are mainly responsible for the laxative effects of senna by increasing fluid secretion and stimulating movement in the gut. Senna also contains naphthalene glycosides. Senna leaves and pods contain small amounts of flavonoids, such as kaempferol and isorharmetin; mucilage, minerals and sugars.

Healing Properties

In 1975, the US Food and Drug Administration (FDA) proposed senna become an over the counter nonprescription laxative. In 1993, the German Commission E approved the use of both "Senna leaf" and "Senna pod" as nonprescription medicines for treating constipation. In 2006 the European Medicines Authority published labelling standards for senna leaf and senna pod as laxatives. Ayurvedic medicine practitioners use Senna leaf for constipation and diseases of the abdomen. Unani medicine uses it for joint pain, backache, hip pain, sciatica, gout, cardiac asthma and several other conditions. Chinese medicine uses senna leaf to treat accumulation of heat marked by constipation and abdominal pain and oedema.

Research

Constipation is common and has many different causes, such as drugs, operations, lack of fibre in the diet, lack of exercise, so several scientists have carried out clinical trials with senna. It's also been investigated as a bowel-preparation method for use before colonoscopy or abdominal imaging. The Natural Standard Research Collaboration (NSRC) published a review in 2011 of all the clinical trials of senna for constipation. In 1973 Greenhalf carried out a single-blind clinical trial of 175 pregnant and breast feeding women, comparing Senokot, a standardised senna preparation to Normacol, a laxative containing Sterculia spp, Frangula spp, powders and decussate sodium. A second study in 1980 compared Senokot to an identical placebo that contained powdered cornflakes and dried grass (!) Unsurprisingly the Senokot worked better at relieving constipation.

Opioids cause constipation. In 1993 Ewe gave loperamide to 24 subjects to cause constipation in the same way as opioids do. Then they compared Sennatin, a senna preparation, Agiocur, which contained psyllium husk and seeds or Agiolax, containing a combination of psyllium and senna. This was a rather small trial but the senna products worked better than the psyllium without the Senna.

Doctors usually give patients polyethyene glycol to clear out the intestines before carrying out surgery on the colon.

In 1999 Valverde carried out a randomised single blind trial of 523 patients with rectal or colonic cancer. He gave polyethylene glycol to half and senna to the other half. He found that the Senna worked better than the polyethylene glycol. In 2005 Radaelli carried a trial on 283 patients preparing for colonoscopy, also comparing senna with polyethylene glycol. He came to the same conclusion, that senna worked better.

Three studies came to the conclusion that the combination of senna with fibre was the more effective than conventional pharmaceutical drugs for constipation.

Part 4

Poisonous Plants in Renaissance Florence

Poisoning was part of the social fabric of Renaissance Italy. In Venice, for example, a Committee of Ten sanctioned poisoning as a tool of government, and kept official records of victims eliminated in this way, according to Smith in 1952. The death penalty by lethal injection in the United States today is similar. The Medici family have long had a reputation as infamous poisoners. But there is little evidence to support this, apart from Cosimo's plot to kill Piero Strozzi in 1548, which he didn't carry out.

Before the eighteenth century it was impossible to tell whether a person had died of poison, as the case of Ferdinando de' Medici, suspected of poisoning his brother Francesco, demonstrates. It was not until 2006 that Fornaciari disproved this poisoning theory. Francesco in fact died of cerebral malaria. Poison mimicked many other ailments and often failed to be fatal. During the Renaissance everyone was suspicious when illustrious people died; and those who believed they were in danger were always wary and suspicious.

Many people, especially men, considered poisoning to be a female crime. In his *Discoverie of Witchcraft* in 1584 Reginald Scot said "women were the first inventors and practisers of the art of poisoning." Italian physician Giovanni Battista Codronchi stated in 1595 that for every one male poisoner there were fifty females. This was all part of the continuing demonisation of women healers, who were not allowed to participate in medical practice, although they had been treating people with their encyclopaedic knowledge of healing plant medicine since time immemorial.

Poison was a major concern for anyone in a position of power or importance. People wrote to Cosimo about suspected poisonings when a sick person or a corpse displayed symptoms such as rashes, bleeding from mouth, nose and ears, vomiting blood, blackened skin and extreme postmortem oedema. Letters to Cosimo stated that Charles IX of France, Cardinal Charles de Lorraine, Countess Bianca Ragnoni Guidi and Cardinal Ippolito de' Medici were all poisoned. Pope Paul III and Henry II of France attempted to poison Ferrante Gonzaga, who in turn conspired with Cosimo to poison Piero Strozzi's wine flask, according to Sheila Barker in 2017. The Medici pope Leo X suffered from severe anal abscesses. Cardinal Petrucci and collaborators plotted to kill him with poisonous bandages applied to his anal ulceration, but the plot was uncovered and the conspirators convicted. When he died in 1521 his cupbearer was accused of poisoning him, was arrested and tried but eventually acquitted. Pope Leo X probably died of disease. The only prominent Medici to die of poisoning was Ippolito, cardinal in Hungary and pawn in the civil strife in Florence, who died in 1535. His assassin, Giovanni Andrea, was subsequently stoned to death in his home town. Cosimo himself was the target of poison plots: in 1556 a letter told him his towels had been poisoned and three years later someone warned him that a trusted woman wanted to poison his food and drink.

The Medici, always aware of the danger of poison, chose their kitchen staff extremely carefully and took all manner of precautions at the dinner table. They used open air salt cellars with silver or gold surfaces because they believed that poison would cause the salt to sweat, and it would be easier to see the droplets of moisture on the shiny surface of the salt cellar. They also thought that salt would counter the effects of the poison, according to Thorndike in 1934. Their wine goblets were fashioned from alexipharmic stones (stones that warded off poison.) Catherine de' Medici gave her granddaughter Christine de Lorraine a green chalcedony cup that would apparently lose its lustre when it came into contact with poison, according to Mercati in 1576. The Mughal Emperor Humayun gave Cosimo I de' Medici a rhinoceros horn cup, for rhinoceros horn was considered a powerful antidote to poison, according to Bacci in 1573. Cosimo was sceptical about the origins of rhinoceros and unicorn horn, but since this was a gift from a Mughal Emperor he reasoned that it should be genuine. Most of the Medici's alexipharmic vessels were made from agate, which was thought to cure scorpion and viper venom, according to Bacci in 1587.

Renaissance Florence abounded in poisonous substances: snake, scorpion, toad and fish venoms, hemlock, black henbane, oleander, aconite, poppy, *nux vomica*, black nightshade, white hellebore; arsenic, gypsum, mercury.

Physicians and apothecaries kept all manner of poisons in locked cupboards, some of which were administered in tiny doses as medicine, such as nightshade as a sleeping drug. Sometimes poison was used for euthanasia, for example, if someone had rabies, an incurable and terribly painful disease. Cosimo I's herbalists in his botanical gardens and at the university in Pisa, could identify all the poisonous plants. The duke of Alba's herbalist made poisons for hunting large game, some of which he sent to Francesco de' Medici. Soldiers coated their knives with poison. Artists worked with highly toxic paints and artisans used poison sumac to make wood varnish. Metallurgists used mercury to refine gold. Monks grew all kinds of poisonous plants in their cloister gardens. The nuns of Santa Petronilla in Perugia poisoned Pope Benedict XI in 1304, according to a manuscript (Magl. XXV, 18) in the National Library of Florence.

Cosimo I's paternal grandmother, Caterina Sforza (1463–1509) left a large collection of alchemical, medical and magical recipes which included some for poisons. In 1566 Cosimo was accused of poisoning his chamberlain Sforza Almeni, though there was never any proof that he did, or indeed that Almeni died of poisoning. In 1548 he sent a letter swearing that he would never think of poisoning anyone and that he didn't possess any relevant recipes. But he lied. He kept a secret poison recipe and he frequented the poison-brewing sorcerer, Apollonio. He also owned several books in which poisons were discussed and his alchemical treatises contained poisonous compositions.

Francesco was an expert toxicologist who recognised that the knife that killed his courtier, Count Clemente Pietro in 1574 was coated with a Spanish poison. Sheila Barker says that Francesco wrote to his agent in Milano in 1590 'A little poison is being sent to you, made just for this purpose. The entire quantity is sufficient to poison a whole flask of wine, and don't use any less, and it is odourless, tasteless and extremely powerful.' Francesco also requested that 'A liquor of venomous plants for killing large animals' be prepared in Madrid in 1575 by the duke of Alva's herbalist. But we have no evidence that he ever used it. After his death, Cosimo's younger son, Ferdinando (1549–1609) was patron to Girolamo Mercuriale, a brilliant toxicologist and author of *De venenis, et morbis venenosis tractatus locupletissimi* in 1584. Ferdinando sent a letter to an agent in 1590, explaining how to put a few drops of poison into the enemy's wine flask, together with a sample of the poison, which he said was odourless, tasteless and highly potent. This sounds to me like arsenic, one of the favourite poisons at the time. A manuscript in the National Library of Florence contains one of Francesco's son, Don Antonio's recipes for a white hellebore root poison "the herb for the cross-bow," (Naz II.I.345.)

But just in case a poisoner should get through all these precautions Cosimo prepared an antidote, from scorpion venom, as previously mentioned. The scorpions were collected in August when their venom was supposed to be mature. He never sold his antidote, but gave it to noblemen who requested it. It was used to treat suspected poisoning, plague, incurable fevers and any other incurable life-threatening condition. He packed it carefully in glass vials within compartments of wooden cases, to prevent degradation and or breakage, according to Sheila Barker in 2017. Antidotes were sometimes tested on condemned criminals and in 1548 Cosimo sent some to duke Ferrante I Gonzaga, recommending that he tried it on a prisoner waiting for capital punishment.

Paracelsus (1493–1541) was the first physician to explain in clear terms that poisons had chemical effects and the severity of these effects depended on the dose taken. Thus certain powerful drugs could be lethal if taken in large doses but therapeutic in smaller doses. The surgeon Ambroise Paré (1510- 1590) contributed towards demystifying the subject of poisoning, and Paulus Zacharias (1584–1659) reviewed existing knowledge of poisons, while disproving that malicious incantations could have a fatal effect.

During the Renaissance many people still believed bull's blood, menstrual blood, nail parings, lobster claws, toad flesh, cat hair, bat hearts and all sorts of other things had mythical poisonous powers, according to Fischer Homberger in 1980. They also believed that all manner of articles of clothing could be poisoned: gloves, slippers, flowers and so on. Many doctors at the time upheld as many superstitions as the people they treated, which only increased the fear of poisoning. I do not believe that the Medici themselves subscribed to any of these superstitions. They were probably using the poisonous plants recorded by Dioscorides: belladonna, henbane, aconite, hellebore, nux vomica, opium, as well as mineral poisons, such as mercury, antimony, lead, copper, arsenic and arsenic derivatives. They may even have used cantharide, ground, dried blister beetle, *Lytta vesicatoria*. They mixed up their poisons in their alchemical laboratories but in most cases I do not think they actually used them. Every great house in Europe at the time had its stock of poisons.

When Francesco's wife, Archduchess Joanna of Austria, died in 1578 and he married his attractive mistress, Bianca Capello, the Florentines turned against their ruler and accused Bianca of possessing the evil eye and poisoning Joanna. Francesco went into seclusion and virtually lived in his alchemical laboratory. This led to further vilification and accusations that he was preparing poisons to be used by the witch, Bianca. When they died simultaneously in October 1587 (of malaria), people assumed that they had been poisoned by Ferdinando or had poisoned themselves. Malaria was endemic in many parts of Italy, especially Maremma, where Francesco liked to go hunting.

Aconite, *Aconitum nepellus*, "the fulgurating exterminator ... was popularised with the Science and Art of the Renaissance," according to Knott in 2014. It belongs to a genus of over two hundred poisonous species. Magister Sautes de Ardoynis listed aconite as a poison in his book of Venoms in 1424, according to Mulvey-Roberts in 2012. It is a member of the Ranunculaceae family and the genus name *Aconitum*, derives from the Greek *akoniton* (without earth) since it can grow on rocky ground. It has blue flowers with five sepals that look like petals. One of these sepals resembles a cylindrical helmet or hood, which is why the English named it monkshood, and it can grow up to one metre on a straight, hairless stalk. People cultivate it in their gardens because it is so beautiful, but its leaves and roots are extremely toxic since it contains the alkaloid, aconitine, which paralyses the heart and nervous system. The roots and root tubers are particularly powerfully poisonous.

In 2021 Alisha Rankin described how in 1524 Gregorio Caravita created a poison antidote which he offered to Pope Clement VII. The Pope commanded his doctors to test it on two criminals who'd been condemned to death. The doctors gave both prisoners a good quantity of aconite, enough to kill "not merely two men but one hundred." As the poison took effect the prisoners screamed in agony as the poison gripped their hearts. Caravita immediately rubbed his antidote oil on one of the men's chests, over his heart and apparently his heart and pulse quickly returned to normal. The second prisoner who was not given the oil died in agony.

However, traditional healers in Asian countries have used aconite as a herbal medicine for its anti-inflammatory and analgesic properties. Tiny amounts stimulate the heart and increase blood flow, improving the digestive system, but accidental poisoning sometimes occurs because the safety margin of the toxic alkaloids is so small, according to Chan in 2012.

According to the Pharmacy historian Julius Berendes in 1891, hellebore (*Veratrum species*) produced the most famous drug in the Greek *Materia Medica* because of its many healing properties. The toxicity of hellebores is mentioned in the Hippocratic writings: "Convulsions following the administration of hellebore are fatal." Hellebores kill, but before doing so they have a few side effects, including nausea and diarrhoea, and since Greek physicians believed in purging their patients they would use hellebore for this purpose. Gerard (1633) in his classical herbal sang the praises of hellebore:

> The root of white Hellebor procureth vomite mightily, wherein consisteth his chief vertue, and by that means voideth all superfluous slimes and naughtie humors.

The Romans knew about *Veratrum album*, (white hellebore) and *Veratrum nigrum*, (black hellebore), which belong to the Melanthiaceae family, and used them as insecticides, according to Klocke in 1989. The root of false white hellebore (*Veratrum album*) contains veratrine alkaloids: potent neurotoxins. As early as the fifth century CE people were coating seeds with extracts of *Veratrum species* before planting, to stop pests from destroying them. This practice continued throughout the

Renaissance. There are several *Veratrum* alkaloids including veratridine, cevadine and veratrine; which all irritate the mucous membranes. Hellebore poisoning causes vomiting, abdominal pain, then slowing down of the heart, low blood pressure and death.

Hemlock (*Conium maculatum*), a member of the Umbelliferae, gains its genus name: *Conium* from the Greek word *Konas*, meaning to whirl about, because if people eat the plant, it causes nausea, vomiting, vertigo followed by death. The species name, *maculatum*, is Latin for spotted, and refers to the stem-markings. The leaves of hemlock are similar to those of many other members of the Umbelliferae, such as the carrot. But the markings on the stem are unique to hemlock. Plato famously described how Socrates was poisoned with hemlock, when he was condemned to death by the law of Athens. Hemlock has a disagreeable mousy smell, especially when it is bruised. The whole plant is poisonous. People have mistakenly eaten the leaves for parsley, the roots for parsnips and the seeds for anise seeds with fatal results. Hemlock contains eight piperidine alkaloids, including the highly toxic gamma-coniceine and coniine.

In Britain farmers are careful to pull up and destroy hemlock plants because if a cow accidentally eats it while pregnant she will give birth to a calf with crooked calf disease. For this reason, hemlock is extremely rare in Britain. However, in Renaissance Florence herbalists, apothecaries, monks and others were growing it to use as a poison and perhaps also as a medicine and in any case, if current practices in Tuscany are anything to go by, cows were not generally left loose to eat what they liked.

Henbane (*Hyoscyamus niger*), is a member of the Solanaceae native to Europe. The Latin binomial is derived from the Greek words *hyos* and *cyamos*, signifying hog's bean, since hogs apparently can eat it with impunity. People have been using henbane as a hallucinogen since time immemorial. Archeologists in Austria dug up an early Bronze Age urn filled with bones, shells and henbane seeds while Assyrian and Babylonian priests used it ritually as a powerful hallucinogen. The Vikings were so keen on henbane that they buried people with hundreds of henbane seeds. Archeologists in Denmark dug up Fyrkat woman who was wearing a pouch of henbane seeds, according to Mrs Grieves. Greek authors, Xenophon and Dioscorides mentioned its intoxicating properties.

During the Renaissance magicians and healers, in the depths of the countryside, far from the eyes of the Florentines, in great secrecy, made henbane concoctions and love philtres. They rubbed flying ointments that contained henbane and other ingredients onto the skin of their armpits, and since atropine, when mixed with fat or oil, was absorbed through the skin, this produced the sensation of flying. Henbane was one of the plants that acted as a bridge to the supernatural. Perger in 1864 wrote:

Witches drank the decoction of henbane and had those dreams for which they were tortured and executed. It was used for witches ointment and ... for making weather and conjuring spirits.

They used it for divination, love magic and as a poison. They smoked leaves in a pipe, believing that it made them invisible. They infused the leaves in oil over a gentle heat to make an erotic massage oil.

In Germany people brewed a psychoactive beer using henbane, which became so popular that gardens of henbane were planted, just for the breweries. This came to an end in 1516 when the Bavarian Purity Laws were introduced. The earliest record of henbane use in Germany was a confessional in 1025:

...they gather several girls and select from these a small maiden as a kind of leader. They disrobe her and take her out of the settlement to a place where they can find *Hyoscyamus,* which is known as bliss in German. They have her pull this out with a little finger of the right hand and tie the uprooted plant to the small toe of the right foot with any kind of string. Then the girls, each of whom is holding a rod in her hands, lead the aforementioned maiden to the next river, pulling the plant behind her. The girls then use the rods to sprinkle the young maiden with river water, and in this way they hope to cause rain through their magic. They take the young maiden, as naked as she is who puts down her feet and moves herself in the manner of a crab, by the hands and lead her from the river back to the settlement.

I doubt that the Florentines were interested in psychoactive beer, being far more interested in their excellent wine.

Dioscorides, who preferred the white henbane, (also called *Veratrum album,*) to other species of henbane which he said could cause madness, soaked the seeds and leaves in hot water and pounded them to create a medicine that would deaden pain and help the patient sleep. Gerard in Chapter 61 of his herbal stated that there were three types of henbane: white, *Hyoscyamus albus*, black, *Hyscyamus niger,* and yellow. In fact Gerard's yellow henbane was tobacco, recently arrived from the Americas. He stated that taking henbane caused drowsiness and assuaged pain but was deadly, and that Pythagoras, Zoroaster, and Apuleius used the name *insana*. Pliny said it was "of the nature of wine and therefore offensive to the understanding." Gerard said:

the leaves, the seeds and the juice (of henbane) cause an unquiet sleep, like unto the sleep of drunkenness, which continues long and is deadly to the patient. To wash the feet in a decoction of henbane as also the often smelling of the flowers causeth sleep.

I was delighted to read that the redoubtable Mrs Grieves described an incident in a monastery where the monks accidentally ate some henbane roots for supper. In the night they began to display a delirious frenzy accompanied by hallucinations, and this continued all through the following day so that the monastery resembled a lunatic asylum. This reminded me of Almodovar's third film, "Dark Habits" ("*Entre Tinieblas*"), set in a nunnery, where each of the nuns is indulging in a different drug and total chaos reigns.

Shakespeare took the name "hebon" (meaning henbane) from Marlow, who mentioned 'hebon" as a deadly poison, when Hamlet's father's Ghost said:

Upon my secure hour thy uncle stole, with juice of cursed hebona in a vial, And in the porches of my ears did pour the leprous distillment, whose effect holds such an enmity with blood of man, that swift as quicksilver it courses through the natural gates and alleys of the body, and with a sudden vigor it doth posset and curd, like eager droppings into milk, the thin and wholesome blood.

Henbane contains tropane alkaloids, including hyoscyamine, hyoscine and scopolamine, plant toxins that occur in several plant families including Solanaceae (e.g. mandrake, henbane, deadly nightshade, Jimson weed,) Erythroxylaceae, Convolvulaceae, Brassicaceae, and Euphorbiaceae. Plants containing tropane alkaloids are some of the world's oldest medicines and people have been using them as analgesics, hallucinogens and poisons for centuries. Tropane alkaloids stop the enzyme cholinesterase from breaking down acetylcholine, which causes the smooth muscles to relax. Hyoscyamine acts on the sweat and salivary glands, heart muscles, stomach, gastrointestinal tract, urinary tract and central nervous system. It lowers blood pressure and heart rate and doctors prescribe to provide relief for gastrointestinal disorders, ulcers, spasms, irritable bowel effects, spastic urinary tract and Parkinson's disease. They give it to patients taking opioid drugs for palliative care to prevent constipation. Adverse side effects include dizziness, dry mucous membranes, irregular heartbeat, tachycardia, flushing, faintness, vomiting, hallucinations, euphoria, disorientation and death. Scopolamine is used to prevent motion sickness.

The school of Salerno in southern Italy produced a collection of formulae called the *Antidotarium parvum* by Nicolas of Salerno probably in the eleventh century, according to Cassar in 1987. This contains a recipe for *spongia somnifera*: an anaesthetic mixture of water, opium, mandrake and henbane, with instructions to soak a rag in it and apply it to the patient's nostrils, to put them to sleep before surgery. Of course, there were people who used henbane potions for more nefarious purposes, such as driving people mad, according to Patricia Aakhus in 2008.

Black nightshade, *Solanum nigrum*, is another member of the Solanaceae, that could have originated in the Middle East or even India, and has been growing in Europe for many centuries, anywhere it can, in waste ground, mixed in with crops and so on. Gerard in his Herbal described and illustrated the garden nightshade and advised that neither the juice nor any part of the plant should be taken internally. The garden nightshade he described is clearly *Solanum nigrum* with:

> leaves of a blackish colour, soft & full of juice, in shape like to the leaves of Basil, but much greater: among which do grow small white flowers with yellow pointels in the middle; which being past, there do succeed rounde berries, greene at the first, and black when they be ripe like those of Jui[c]e: the roote is white and full of hairie strings.

Solanum nigrum appears in Dioscorides' Materia Medica as well as various Renaissance sources. The whole plant contains the toxic tropane glyco-alkaloid solanine, but the unripe berries have the highest concentration of it. When the berries are ripe they contain less solanine than the rest of the plant, according to Cooper and Johnson in 1984. Solanine is toxic in minute quantities. Black nightshade poisoning causes nausea, vomiting, diarrhoea, headache, dizziness, loss of speech, fever, sweating, irregular heartbeat, pupil dilation, blindness, mental confusion, convulsions, coma, and death. However, traditional healers in India have been using it for its anti-inflammatory, anti-seizure, anti-oxidant, antiviral properties and to protect the liver according to Reema Gabrani in 2012. Black nightshade was used as a poison in Renaissance Florence, but it may also have been used as a medicine.

Thorn apple or Jimson weed, *Datura stramonium*, native to the Americas, is another member of the Solanaceae. People have been smoking the dried plant as a hallucinogen for centuries, according to Williams in 2013. Gerard in Chapter 57 of his Herbal describes two Datura species, *D. metel* L. ("round fruite full of short and blunt prickles") and Jimson weed, *Datura stramonium* ("the fruit ... rounde, sometimes of the fashion of an egge, set about on every part with most sharpe prickles"), both plants from the Americas.

All parts of the plant contain toxic tropane alkaoids. Poisoning causes dry mouth, blurred vision, photophobia, irregular heartbeat, flushing, jerking movements, short term memory loss, disorientation, confusion, hallucinations, psychosis, agitated delirium, seizures, coma, inability to breathe and heart attack. However, traditional healers have been using it for its anti-epileptic, anti-asthmatic, analgesic, antioxidant, antimicrobial and insecticidal properties, according to Al-Snafi in 2017. This is yet another plant that was used as a poison in Renaissance Florence, but may also have been used as a medicine.

Mandrake, *Mandragora officinalis*, is yet another member of the Solanaceae. Gerard in Chapter 60 of his herbal described it and discussed, the male and female forms (shown later to be different species) on the basis of fruit shape and leaf colour. He poured scorn on the ridiculous "old wives" tales about the plant shrieking when it was dug up and stated that he and his servants frequently dug and replanted it. He described the many medicinal properties of the plant, including its soporific effect and the way it rendered sterile women fertile. However, he covered himself by quoting Psalm 127:3, that:

Children and the fruite of the womb are the inheritaunce, that commeth from the Lord.

Shakespeare's Cleopatra says:

Give me to drink mandragora. ...
That I might sleep out this great gap of time my Antony is away.

The opium poppy, whose Latin binomial, *Papaver somniferum*, means the "sleep-bringing poppy," is the king of medicinal plants, containing a veritable cornucopia of active compounds, which can be used by health professionals for a multitude of medical needs. The World Health Organisation lists medicines derived from the opium poppy as essential drugs, because they provide the most effective pain relief.

Dioscorides provided detailed instructions on making opium, as well as how to detect adulterations and imitations of the drug. He pounded the poppy heads with the leaves, pressed them, crushed them in a mortar with pestle and made pills out of the resultant paste. According to him a pill the size of a small pea would relieve suffering, bring sleep and comfort in the case of long illnesses but excessive consumption would eventually kill the patient. Florentine physicians, who followed the writings of Dioscorides, would have prepared opium in the same way.

The opium poppy may have done as much damage to humanity as good, due to its addictive properties. For a full description of the Opium Wars in China, see my book: *Healing plants of the Celtic Druids.*

Oleander: *Nerium oleander* belongs to the Apocynaceae family, native to the Mediterranean and grown as an ornamental plant worldwide. All parts of this plant are toxic and contain a variety of cardiac glycosides including nerifolin and oleandrin. It was considered a valuable medicinal plant in ancient times, according to Kawalekar in 2012. People have been using oleander leaves, leaf juice and bark latex to treat diseases caused by fungi and bacteria, as well as warts and ulcers for centuries. It was used as a remedy against cancer in the Middle Ages, according to Haux in 1999. Doctors used to prescribe cardiac glycosides for treating heart failure and certain irregular heartbeats, but now less and less since it is so difficult to measure the exact dosage needed. Cardiac glycoside overdose results in blurred vision, seeing yellow, green and white haloes round things, rash, diarrhoea, nausea, vomiting, stomach pain, irregular or slow heartbeat, low blood pressure, weakness, confusion, depression, drowsiness, fainting, hallucinations, headache and death.

Strychnos nux-vomica L., a deciduous tree, belongs to the genus *Strychnos* of the Loganiaceae family and grows in Sri Lanka, India, Vietnam, Thailand, Cambodia and Malaysia. European countries, including Italy, began to use it in the sixteenth century to poison dogs, cats, crows and other animals, according to Williams in 2009. The most famous alkaloid in *nux vomica* is strychnine, which is violently poisonous to the cerebrospinal system. 0.259g of strychnine is fatal. In about an hour the poisoned person starts to feel as if they are suffocating, then all the muscles of the body convulse violently, they fling their arms and legs out, clench their hands, jerk their head forwards and backwards for a minute or two. The muscles relax for a couple of minutes then the convulsions start again and again there is a brief pause, after which the convulsions become more and more severe, until the poisoned person is bent into a bow, their head and heels on the ground, abdominal muscles as hard as a board, and eyeballs staring. In the end they die of exhaustion and asphyxiation, according to Justice in 2012.

Physicians in the countries where *Strychnos nux-vomica* is native use the seed for its analgesic and anti-inflammatory actions, its anti-tumour and immune system regulatory effects and its ability to inhibit pathogens, according to Guo in 2018. It contains alkaloids, iridoid and flavonoid glycosides, triterpenoids, steroids and organic acids, among other compounds. Some people even chew the seeds for their aphrodisiac properties, according to Dutta in 1980.

Conclusions

The Renaissance was a period of unparalleled beauty, excitement and interest in Florence, despite frequent plagues and wars, thanks in large part to the presence of the Medici family, who virtually invented modern banking and accountancy. They tapped into foreign trade networks, providing letters of foreign exchange and soon became the richest family in Europe. They were outstanding as enlightened and successful patrons of art, architecture, science, philosophy and above all, every aspect of plant medicine. They collected medicinal and rare plants, created large gardens around their villas and botanic gardens which are still there today.

Unlike billionaires of today, they did not believe in saving and storing their money but spent it almost as fast as they made it, (even faster, in the case of Lorenzo the Magnificent.) The cream of the artistic world flooded into Florence to seek the patronage of the great Medici family.

This was a time when the whole world was changing, due to numerous voyages of exploration. Medicinal, food and decorative plants were being transported across the world and transplanted into countries where they had never grown before. The Medici were as excited as everyone else by the new plants, and they had the means to acquire them and grow them in their botanic gardens. Plants such as maize, sunflower and tomato from south America were to become staple crops in Italy, while citrus fruits from India and south east Asia also made their way to Italy, were transplanted and adopted. Cosimo I was so interested in these voyages of exploration that he commissioned numerous maps, and Florence became a centre of geographical and cartographical research.

The Medici patronage of the University of Pisa, Cosimo I's creation of the chair of simples (medicinal plants) and his employment of Luca Ghini, revolutionised the way that herbal medicine was taught. No longer a theoretical discipline in which the doctors had no knowledge of the plants used in their medicine, the study of plants was to become integral to the study of medicine and herbal medicine became a discipline that was taken seriously. Francesco's employment of Cesalpino in the chair of simples led to his collection of dried specimens of all the medicinal plants, and to the creation of the first herbarium. This was yet another major step forward in the accurate identification of medicinal plants and herbaria are now universally adopted.

The Medici were responsible for collecting ancient herbal treatises, such as Dioscorides De Materia Medica, and promoting their translation into the vernacular. Cosimo's patronage of Mattioli led to the production of the most famous herbal of the time, with accurate botanical drawings. Although the fathers of botanical art, above all Fuchs, resided in Germany, it was the Medici patronage of botanists and artists that helped to disseminate botanical knowledge. Seeds, dried specimens and accurate drawings and paintings of plants were exchanged and plant knowledge spread outwards in ever increasing circles from Florence and its associated University in Pisa.

Their patronage of alchemy resulted in many useful discoveries, such as the creation of artists' pigments, compounded dyes for the cloth industry, and better distillation techniques for medicinal plants. Alchemy had a profound influence on literature, poetry, fine art and philosophy, and especially chemistry. Marsilio Ficino incorporated alchemical ideas into his philosophy of humanism, which focussed primarily on what it was to be human, within a Christian/neo-Platonic framework. Despite living in an age of war, plague and syphilis, humanism was supremely optimistic, based on the idea of a rebirth of classical culture. It had a tremendous impact on all aspects of life in Renaissance Italy, from government to the arts, and later on the rest of Europe.

And while the Medici family were busy promoting art, culture, science, philosophy and herbal medicine in Florence they were also keeping the warring states of Milan, Naples and Rome at bay, no easy task at a time when everyone was at each other's throats and even the Pope was throwing his weight about.

References

Introduction

Acton H 1979. The Pazzi Conspiracy: The plot against the Medici. Southampton: The Camelot Press.

Aldrovani Bibliotecca del Universita di Bologna MS 136 vol 14. Catalogus omnium plantarum qua erant in horto publico studiorum tempore Luca Gini qui publice profitebatur lectionem simplicium, et horti studiorum praefectus erat.

Ames-Lewis F 1984. The Library and Manuscripts of Piero di Cosimo de' Medici. New York.

Archivio di Stato di Firenze, Guardaroba Medicea, 228 ins. 6, c. 582

Bacci and Forlani. Mostra di disegni di Jacopo Ligozzi. p 21.

Baldini B 1578. Vita di Cosimo I il Granduca di Toscana. Florence Bartolomeo Sermatelli. p 86–87.

Ball P 2001. Bright Earth: The Invention of Colour. Penguin.

Barker S 2015. Renaissance Society of America Annual Conference in Berlin entitled "The Grand Duke's Medicinal Secrets: Pharmacy at the Medici Court, 1600–1630."

Barker S 2016. The Contributions of Medici Women to Medicine in Grand Ducal Tuscany and Beyond. In The Grand Ducal Medici and their Archive 1537–1743, ed Alessio Assonitis and Brian Sandberg (Turnhout), 101–116, 103, 105.

Barker S 2021. Cosimo i de' Medici and the Renaissance Sciences: "To Measure and to See." Brill's Companion to Cosimo I de Medici ed A Assonitis and H Th van Veen.

bncf, Magliabechiano, xv, 111.

Belon P. Les remonstrances sur le default du labour and culture des plants et de la connaissance d'icelles. Paris 1558; ch 22. La grand beauté dont le jardin de Castello du Florence est orné pp 79v–80r.

Bencivvenni Pelli, Descrizione della Galleria di Filippo Pigafetta p 199.

"Book in which will be written experiments and reliable things [made] by the hand of the duke of Florence, or otherwise in his presence, nor will there be anything that is not absolutely proven for the common good". bncf, Palatino 1139.

The Botany of Leonardo da Vinci. A vision of science bridging art and nature. Florence Santa Maria. Novella Museum. 13 September–15 November 2019.

Butters S 1996. The Triumph of Vulcan: Sculptors' Tools, Porpyry and the Prince in Ducal Florence, 2 vols. Florence ch 14, pp 241–67.

Campanelli M 2019. Marsilio Ficino's portrait of Hermes Trismegistus and its afterlife. Intellectual History Review; 29(1): 53–71. From ancient theology to civil religion.

Cennino Cennini 1390. Il libro dell'arte (The Craftsman's Handbook), transl. D. V. Thompson Dover, New York, 1960.

Cinelli G Bozze Delle bellezze di Firenze. BNCF Magliab XIII.

Concini B (collector) Segreti diversi, bncf, Magl xvi, 34, fols 110v, 241r.

Corrias A 2012. Imagination and Memory in Marsilio Ficino's Theory of the Vehicles of the Soul. Internat J of the Platonic Tradition 6; 81–114. 2012.

Crisciani C 1996. Cited by Crisciani in: Opus and sermo: The Relationship between Alchemy and Prophecy (12th–14th Centuries) Early Science and Medicine 13(1); 4–24253.

Dante, Divina Commedia, Inferno XXIX, 118–20, 136–9.

De Thermis Andreae Baccii Elpidiani, Medici atque Philosophi, civis Romanis, Libri septem, Venezia 1571 ch 8 p 370. Quoted by Perifano, Al'Alchimie. P111.

Dibernard B 1977. Kunstkammer (The Golden Fleece 1598–1599) Julius Khon, 44. 274–289 London 1920 (appendix) George Ripley 1591.

El ricettario dell'arte, et università de' medici, et spetiali della città di Firenze (Florence: 1550), 6–7.

Fedeli V. Relazione di Firenze di Messer Vincenzo Fedeli tornato da quella corte l'anno 1561; in *Relazioni degli ambasciatori veneti al senato*, ed. Eugenio Albèri, 15 vols (Florence: 1839–1863), ser. ii, vol. i, 356.

Ferrini V 1173. Letter of 2 April; Archivio di Stato Firenze, Medici del Principato, 1173, c. 142.

Findlen P 1999. The formation of a scientific community; natural history in sixteenth century Italy, in Anthony Grafton and Nancy Siraisi (eds), Natural Particulars; nature and the disciplines in Renaissance Europe. Cambridge MA; 369–400.

Galluzzi R 1781. Istoria del Granducato di Toscana sotto il governo di casa Medici. Florence. P 294.

Galluzzi P 1980. I Medici protettori delle scienze: Tra mito e realtà," in *La corte* (Milan: 1980), 131, and cat. entry 5.20, 174–175.

Greene EL and Egerton FN Ed 1983. Landmarks of Botanical History p 718. Stanford.

Hedesan G 2022. Medical Alchemy in Renaissance Florence. Transforming Materials at Palazzo Vecchio and Casino di San Marco. Institutio Santariana. Fondazione Comel.

Kieffer F 2014. The laboratories of Art and Alchemy at the Uffizi Gallery in Renaissance Florence: Some material Aspects. In: Laboratories of Art: Alchemy and art technology from antiquity to the eighteenth century by Dupre S.

Klein U and Eddy MD Eds 2022. The core concepts and cultural context of eighteenth century chemistry. A cultural History of chemistry in the eighteenth century. London: Bloomsbury. 1–21.

Laguna A 1555. Pedacio Dioscorides Anazarbeo, acerca de la materia medicinal y de los venenos mortiferos (Antwerp) liber iv, ch. 105, 443.

Lapini A. Diario fiorentino di Agostino alpini: dal 252 al 1596, ora per la prima volta pubblicato da GO Corazini. Florence 1900; 107.

Lazzero, The Italian Renaissance Garden p 61.

Letter of an unknown correspondent to Cosimo I, 5 March 1549 in asf, Mediceo del Principato 12, fol. 334r (map doc id# 20927.)

Lippi D 2017. Acromegaly in Lorenzo the Magnificent, father of the Renaissance. The Lancet. Correspondence 389; 10084; 2104.

Maier M 1618. Atlanta fugiens, Oppenheim, J. Th. de Bry.

Marinozzi S et al 2015. Baccio Baldini (1517–1589), Protomedico alla corte medicea tra umanesimo e sperimentalismo. Acta Medico-Historica Adriatica 13/2; 354–364, 357–358.

Marzi D 1896. *La questione della riforma del calendario* (Florence: 1896), 149–167.

Merrifield MP 1849. 59. Recipe no 26.

Mino G 1997. 143–165.

Nardi GB, bncf, Magliabechi- ano, xv, 142.

Orlandi GL Cosimo e Francesco de Medici alchimisti. Florence 1978.

Parisiensis C, *L'Aspertorio Alfabeticale* [...] bncf, Palatino 203.

Perifano, in L' Alchimie à la Cour de Côme ier de Médicis, 58–59.

Plaisance M 1974–1975. *Culture et politique à Florence de* 1542 *à* 1551; in *Les écrivains et le pouvoir en Italie à l' époque de la Renaissance*, ed. André Rochon, 2 vols (Paris: 1974–1975), vol. 1, 153 Poliziano A. *Coniurationis commentarium* / Commentario della congiura dei Pazzi. Firenze Uni Press.

Pratilli GC 1975. *L'università e il principe* (Florence: 1975), 119–135.

Rupescissa 1561. De consideratione quintæ essentiæ (Basle, 1561).

Sandri L 2012. Il Collegio medico fiorentino e la rifoma di Cosimo i: Origini e funzione (sec. xiv–xvi)," in Umanesimo e università in Toscana (1300–1600), ed. Stefano U. Baldassarri,

Fabrizio Ricciardelli, and Enrico Spagnesi (Florence: 2012), 183–211, 195–196, 206.

Seybold S 1990. Luca Ghini, Leonhard Rauwolf und Leonhart Fuchs. Uber die Herkunft der Aquarelle im Wiener Krauterbuchmanuskrpt von Fuchs, Jahresheft der Gesellschaft fur die Naturkunde in Württemberg. Stuttgart 239–326.

Smith P 2004. Note 36, 141, 142.

Stephenson HD 2015. Unlucky in affairs of business... Turning Points in the life of Lorenzo de Medici. Masters Degree from Duke Uni.

Tedaldi GB. "Discorso dell'agricoltura," bncf, Magliabechiano, xiv, 14.

Thompson DV 1956. The Materials and Techniques of Medieval Painting. Dover, New York.

Thorndike L 1923–58. A history of magic and experimental science, vol 6, chap 40 Cesapino's view of nature pp 325–38.

Tozzetti T, "Le Selve," vi, 13: "per bene imprimere nella memoria le fattezze."

Varchi B, "Lezzione nella quale si disputa della maggioranza delle arti e quale sia la più nobile, la sculturao la pittura," *Disputaii* (1546), in *Trattatid'arte del Cinque cento fra Manierismo e Controriforma*, ed. Paola Barocchi, 3 vols (Bari: 1960–1962), vol. 1, 39: "grandissima utilità nelle scienze."

Vasari G, Le vite de' più eccellenti pittori, scultori et architettori, ed. Gaetani Milanesi (Florence: 1878–1885), vol. 6, 544.

Vasari G, Vita di Niccolò detto il Tribolo in Le vote. Novara 1967, vol 5; 443–84. Azzi Vicentini ed, L'Arte dei Giardini.

Water, Gardens, and Hydraulics in Sixteenth-Century Florence and Naples," in *Technology and the Garden*, ed. Michael G. Lee and Kenneth I. Helphand (Washington, DC: 2014), 129–153.

Ziolkowski T 2015. Souls on Wing. Chapter II. 48.

Part 2 Healing Plants of the Renaissance

Archivio dell'ospedale degli Innocenti, Fondo Estranei. Firenze.

Bellorini C 2016. The world of plants in Renaissance Tuscany. Medicine and Botany. Routledge.

Il ricettario medicinale necessario a tutti i medici, e speziali. Florence 1567.

Mattioli, Discorsi 1568.

Chapter 1 Aloe *Aloe vera*

Aloe vera drawing from Kadanaku (in Malayalam); vol. 11, plate 3 Page URL: [1] 11–3 Rheede 1692.png.

American Botanical Council 2016. Systematic Review of the bioactive components and clinical effects of *Aloe vera* gel. HerbClip Issue 539.

American Botanical Council 2016. Herbalgram. Issue 87. Page 1–5 by Gayle Engels.

Bystrom LM 2016. Systematic Review of the Bioactive Components and Clinical Effects of *Aloe Vera* Gel. American Botanical Council. HerbClip 081513–539.

Hakmatpou D, Mehrabi F et al 2019. The Effect of *Aloe Vera* Clinical Trials on Prevention and Healing of Skin Wound: A Systematic Review. Iran J Med Sci 44 (1) PMC 6330525.

Chapter 2 Aniseed *Pimpinella anisum*

Aniseed drawing by the author Angela Paine.

Akhtar A et al 2008. *In vitro* antibacterial activity of *Pimpinella anisum* fruit extracts against some pathogenic bacteria. Veterinary World 1(9): 272–274.

Ashraffodin Ghoshegir S et al 2015. *Pimpinella anisum* in the treatment of functional dyspepsia: A double-blind, randomised clinical trial. J Res Med Sci 20(1): 13–21.

Besharati-Seidani A et al 2005. Headspace solvent micro extraction: a very rapid method for identification of volatile components of Iranian *Pimpinella anisum* seed. Analytica Chimica Acta. 530 (1): 155–161.

Farahmand M et al 2019. Could Anise decrease the intensity of premenstrual syndrome symptoms in comparison to placebo? A double-blind randomised clinical trial. J Comp Integrat Med. https://doi.org/10.1515/jcim-2019–0077.

Hamdollah Mosavata Abbas et al 2019. Efficacy of Anise (*Pimpinella anisum* L) oil for migraine headache: A pilot randomised placebo-controlled clinical trial. J Ethnopharmacol 236: 155–160.

Mosaffa-Jahromi et al 2016. Efficacy and safety of enteric coated capsules of anise oil to treat irritable bowel syndrome. J Ethnopharmacol 194: 937–946.

Nahidi F et al 2008. Effect of Anise extract on hot flush of menopause. Pajoohandeh 13(3): 167–173.

Rajab A 2016. Comparative Study of Physical and Chemical Properties of the Oil Extracted from Fresh and Storage Aniseed and Determination of the Optimal Extraction Method. Internat J Asie Shojaii and Mehri Abdollahi Fard 2012. Review of Pharmacological Properties and Chemical Constituents of *Pimpinella anisum*. Pharmacog and Phytochem Res; 8(9); 1465–1470.

Singletary KW 2002. Anise. Potential health benefits. Nutrition Today 3/4. 57 (2): 96–109.

Chapter 3 Chamomile *Matricaria chamomilla and Chamomilla recutita*

Chamomile drawing from Kohler Medizin Pflanzen 1897.

Albring M et al 1983. The measuring of the anti-inflammatory effect of a compound on the skin of volunteers. Meth Find Exp Clin Pharmacol; 5: 75–77.

Amsterdam JD et al 2009. A randomized, double-blind, placebo-controlled trial of oral *Matricaria recutita* (Chamomile) extract therapy for generalized anxiety disorder. J Clin Psychopharmacol; 29: 378–382.

Birt DF et al 1997. Pinch HC. Inhibition of ultraviolet light induced skin carcinogenesis in SKH-1 mice by apigenin, a plant flavonoid. Anticancer Res; 17: 85–91.

Cemek M et al 2008. Antihyperglycemic and antooxidative potential of *Matricaria chamomilla* L. in streptozotocin-induced diabetic rats. J. Nat Med; 62: 284–293.

Evans S et al 2009. The effect of a novel botanical agent TBS-101 on invasive prostate cancer in animal models. Anti-Cancer Res; 10: 3917–3924.

Gardiner P 2007. Complementary, Holistic, and Integrative Medicine: Chamomile. Pediatr Rev; 28: 16–18.

Gates MA et al 2007. A prospective study of dietary flavonoid intake and incidence of epithelial ovarian cancer. Int. J Cancer; 121: 2225–2232.

Glowania HJ et al 1987. Effect of chamomile on wound healing–a clinical double-blind study. Z Hautkr; 62: 1267–1271.

Gould L et al 1973. Cardiac effects of chamomile tea. J Clin Pharmacol; 11: 475–479.

Hertog MG et al 1993. Dietary antioxidant flavonoids and risk of coronary heart disease: the Zutphen Elderly Study. Lancet. 342: 1007–1011.

Kato A et al 2008. Protective effects of dietary chamomile tea on diabetic complications. J Agric Food Chem; 56: 8206–8211.

Khayyal MT et al 2006. Mechanisms involved in the gastro-protective effect of STW 5 (Iberogast) and its components against ulcers and rebound acidity. Phytomedicine; 13: 56–66.

Kell T. More on infant colic. *Birth Gaz.* 1997; 13:3.

Kroll U and Cordes C 2006. Pharmaceutical prerequisites for a multi-target therapy. Phytomedicine; 5: 12–19.

Lyseng-Williamson KA and Perry CM 2003. Micronised purified flavonoid fraction: a review of its use in chronic venous insufficiency, venous ulcers, and haemorrhoids. Drugs; 63: 71–100.

Martins MD et al 2009. Comparative analysis between *Chamomilla recutita* and corticosteroids on wound healing. An *in vitro* and *in vivo* study. Phytother Res; 23: 274–278.

Mattioli Discorsi 1568. Ch 121; 535–9.

Merfort I et al 1994. In vivo skin penetration studies of camomile flavones. *Pharmazie*; 49:509–511.

Nayak BS et al 2007. Wound healing activity of *Matricaria recutita* L. extract. J Wound Care; 16: 298–302.

Nissen HP et al 1988. Prolifometrie, eine methode zur beurteilung der therapeutischen wirsamkeit kon Kamillosan®-Salbe. Z Hautkr; 63: 84–90.

Paladini AC et al 1999. Flavonoids and the central nervous system: from forgotten factors to potent anxiolytic compounds. J Pharm Pharmacol; 51: 519–526.

Patzelt-Wenczler R and Ponce-Pöschl E 2000. Proof of efficacy of Kamillosan(R) cream in atopic eczema. Eur. J Med Res; 5: 171–175.

Saller R et al 1990. Dose dependency of symptomatic relief of complaints by chamomile steam inhalation in patients with common cold. Eur J Pharmacol; 183: 728–729.

Shinomiya K et al 2005. Hypnotic activities of chamomile and passiflora extracts in sleep-disturbed rats. Biol Pharm Bull; 28: 808–810.

Srivastava JK and Gupta S 2007. Antiproliferative and apoptotic effects of chamomile extract in various human cancer cells. J Agric Food Chem; 55: 9470–9478.

Wang Y et al 2005. A metabonomic strategy for the detection of the metabolic effects of chamomile (*Matricaria recutita* L.) ingestion. J Agric Food Chem; 53: 191–196.

Way TD et al 2004. Apigenin induces apoptosis through proteasomal degradation of HER2/neu in HER2/neu-overexpressing breast cancer cells via the phosphatidylinositol-3′-kinase/Akt-dependent pathway. J Biol Chem; 279: 4479–4489.

Chapter 4 Carob Tree *Ceratonia siliqua*

Drawing of carob by the author, Angela Paine.

Agrawal A et al 2011. Carob (*Ceratonia siliqua*): Health, Medicine and Chemistry. Nat. Prod. Res., 2011, 25, 450–456.

Amessis-Ouchemoukh N 2017. Bioactive metabolites involved in the antioxidant, anti-cancer and anticalpain activities of *Ficus carica* L; *Ceratonia siliqua* L and *Quercus ilex* extracts. Industrial Crops and Products 95; 6–17.

Berrougui H et al 2008. Chem. Phys. Lipids, 2008, 154, S53-S54.

Beynon D 1949. Arobon in the Treatment of Infantile Gastro-Enteritis: A Clinical Trial. Arch Dis Child. 24(117): 41–44.

Corsi L 2002. Antiproliferative effects of *Ceratonia siliqua* L. On mouse hepatocellular carcinoma cell line. Fitoterapia 73(7–8); 674–84.

Forestieri AM et al 1989. Effects of Guar and Carob Gums on Glucose, Insulin and Cholesterol Plasma Levels in the Rat. Phytother. Res. 3, 1–4.

Jaffari H et al 2020. The Effect of 8 Weeks of Carob Supplementation and Resistance Training on Lipid Profile and Irisin in Obese Men. IJSEHR; 4, 91–95.

Kumazawa S et al 2002. Antioxidant activity of polyphenols in carob pods. J Agric Food Chem. 16; 50(2); 373–7.

Macho-Gonzalez et al 2017. Fibre purified extracts of carob fruit decrease carbohydrate absorption. J Food Funct. 8; 2258–2265.

Macho-González A et al 2019. Can Carob-Fruit-Extract-Enriched Meat Improve the Lipoprotein Profile, VLDL-Oxidation, and LDL Receptor Levels Induced by an Atherogenic Diet in STZ-NAD-Diabetic Rats? Nutrients 11, 332.

Macho-González A et al 2020. Carob-Fruit-Extract-Enriched Meat Modulates Lipoprotein Metabolism and Insulin Signalling in Diabetic Rats Induced by High-Saturated-Fat Diet. J. Funct. Foods 64, 103600.

Mokhtari M 2011. The Effect of Hydro - Alcoholic Seeds Extract of *Ceratonia siliqua* on the Blood Glucose and Lipids Concentration in Diabetic Male Rats. International Conference on Life Science and Technology IPCBEE vol.3 (2011) © (2011) IACSIT Press, Singapore.

Papakonstantinou, E et al 2017. Short-Term Effects of a Low Glycemic Index Carob-Containing Snack on Energy Intake, Satiety, and Glycemic Response in Normal-Weight, Healthy Adults: Results from Two Randomized Trials. Nutrition, 42, 12–19.

Zunft HJ et al 2003. Carob Pulp Preparation Rich in Insoluble Fibre Lowers Total and LDL Cholesterol in Hypercholesterolemic Patients. Eur J Nutr 42, 235–242.

Chapter 5 Coriander *Coriandrum sativum*

Coriander drawing: Wellcome M0015406.jpg.

Abascal K and Yarnell E 2012. Cilantro - culinary herb or miracle medicinal plant? Altern Complement Ther; 18(5):259–264.

Aissaoui A et al 2011. Hypoglycemic and hypolipidemic effects of *Coriandrum sativum* L. in meriones shawi rats. J Ethnopharmacol. 2011; 137:652–661.

Ashraf R et al 2020. Cold pressed coriander (*Coriandrum sativum*) seed oil. In Cold Pressed Oils. Green Technology, Bioactive Compounds, Functionality and Applications; 345–356.

Dhanapakiam P et al 2008. The cholesterol lowering property of coriander seeds (*Coriandrum sativum*): Mechanism of action. J Environ Biol; 29(1):53–56.

Eidi M and Eidi A 2011. Effect of coriander (*Coriandrum sativum*) seed ethanol extract in experimental diabetes. Nuts and Seeds in Health and Disease Prevention; 395–400.

Emamghoreishi M and Heldari-Hamedani G 2006. Sedative-hypnotic activity of extracts and essential oil of coriander seeds. Iran J Med Sci;31(1):22–27.

Mandal S and Mandal M 2015. Coriander (*Coriandrum sativum* L) essential oil: chemistry and biological activity. Asian Pacific J Trop Biomed. 5(6):421–428.

Mansour A et al 2015. Effect of coriander fruit on clinical course of migraine patients: a comparison between random effect and transition models. Intern Med Today 21(2): 129–134.

Momin AH et al 2012. *Coriandrum sativum* — review of advances in phytopharmacology. Int J Pharm Sci Res; 5:1233.

Nadeem M 2013. Nutritional and medicinal aspects of coriander (*Coriandrum sativum*): A review. British Food Journal; 115(5):743–755.

Nakamura A et al 2009. Stress repression in restrained rats by (R)-(–)-linalool inhalation and gene expression profiling of their whole blood cells. J Agric Food Chem; 57(12):5480–5485.

Pandey A et al 2011. Pharmacological screening of *Coriandrum sativum* linn. for hepatoprotective activity. J Pharm & Bioallied Sci; 3(3):435–441.

Rajeshwari CU et al 2012. Original article: Antioxidant and anti-arthritic potential of coriander (*Coriandrum sativum* L.) leaves. e-SPEN Journal.;7:e223-e228.

Chapter 6 Dill *Anethum graveolens*

Drawing of dill by the author.

Babri RA et al 2012. Chemical composition and insecticidal activity of the essential oil of *Anethum graveolens*. L. Sci Int (Lahore) 24(4): 453–455.

Goodarzi MT 2016. The role of *Anethum graveolens* L (Dill) in the management of diabetes. J Trop Med published online doi: 10.1155/2016/1098916.

Haidari F et al 2020. The effects of *Anethum graveolens* (dill) powder supplementation on clinical and metabolic status in patients with type 2 diabetes. Trials 21: 483.

Heidarifar R et al 2014. Effect of Dill (*Anthem graveolens*) on the severity of primary dysmenorrhea in comparison with mefenamic acid: A randomised double-blind trial. J Res Med Sci 19 (4): 326–330.

Jalili C et al 2021. Effects of *Anethem graveolens* (dill) and its derivatives on controlling cardiovascular risk factors: A systematic review and meta-analysis. J Herbal Med 30, 100516.

Jana S and Shekhawat GS 2010. *Anethum graveolens:* An Indian traditional medicinal herb and spice. Pharmacy Rev 4(8): 179–184.

Naseri-Gharib MK and Heidari A 2007. Antispasmodic effect of *A graveolens* fruit extract on rat ileum. Int J Pharm 3: 260–4.

Yazdanparast R and Bahramikia S 2007. Improvement of liver antioxidant status in hypercholesterolamic rats treated with *A graveolens* extracts. Pharmacologyonline. 2007;3: 88–94.

Chapter 7 Fennel *Foeniculum vulgare*

Drawing of fennel by the author.

Akgül A and Bayrak A 1988. Comparative volatile oil composition of various parts from Turkish bitter fennel (*Foeniculum vulgare* var. *vulgare*) Food Chemistry 30(4):319–323.

Akha O et al 2014. The effect of fennel (*Foeniculum vulgare*) gel 3% in decreasing hair thickness in idiopathic mild to moderate hirsutism, a randomized placebo controlled clinical trial. Caspian J Intern Med. 2014; 5:26–29.

Albert-Puleo M 1980. Fennel and anise as estrogenic agents. J Ethnopharmacol; 2(4):337–344.

Bokaie M et al 2013. Oral fennel (*Foeniculum vulgare*) drop effect on primary dysmenorrhea: effectiveness of herbal drug. Iran J Nurs Midwifery Res; 18:128–132.

Choi E and Hwang J 2004. Anti-inflammatory, analgesic and antioxidant activities of the fruit of *Foeniculum vulgare*. Fitoterapia; 75(6):557–565.

Duško BL et al 2006. Antibacterial activity of some plants from family Apiaceae in relation to selected phytopathogenic bacteria. Kragujevac Journal of Science; 28:65–72.

Ghazanfarpour M et al 2018. Double-blind, placebo-controlled trial of Fennel (*Foeniculum vulgare*) on menopausal symptoms: a high placebo response. J Turk Ger Gynecol Assoc; 19:122–127.

Khorshidi N et al 2003. Clinical effects of fennel essential oil on primary dysmenorrhea. Iran J Pharm Res; 2:89–93.

Kian FR et al 2017. Evaluating the effect of fennel soft capsules on the quality of life and its different aspects in menopausal women: a randomized clinical trial. Nurs Pract Today; 4:87–95.

Kim, Sang-Moo et al 2008. The Anticaries Activity of Hot Water Extracts from *Foeniculum vulgare*. Applied Biological Chemistry 51; 1:84–87. 2468–0834(pISSN) / 2468–0842(eISSN).

Koppula S and Kumar H 2013. *Foeniculum vulgare* Mill (Umbelliferae) attenuates stress and improves memory in wister rats. Tropical Journal of Pharmaceutical Research; 12(4):553–558.

Mohaddese M 2019. *Foeniculum vulgare* as valuable plant in management of women's health. J Menopausal Med; 25(1): 1–14.

Martins MR, et al 2012. Chemical composition, antioxidant and antimicrobial properties of three essential oils from Portuguese flora. Journal of Pharmacognosy; 3(3):39–44.

Naga Kishore R et al 2012. Evaluation of anxiolytic activity of ethanolic extract of *Foeniculum vulgare* in mice model.

International Journal of Pharmacy and Pharmaceutical Sciences; 4(3):584–586.

Nassar MI et al 2010. Secondary metabolites and pharmacology of *Foeniculum vulgare* Mill. Subsp. *Piperitum*. Revista Latinoamericana de Química; 38(2):103–112.

Nazarpour S and Azimi H 2007. Comparison of therapeutic effects of fennelin and mefenamic acid on primary dysmenorrhea. J Mazandaran Univ Med Sci.; 17:54–61.

Omidali F 2015. The effect of Pilates exercise and consuming Fennel on pre-menstrual syndrome symptoms in non-athletic girls. Complement Med J Fac Nurs Midwifery; 5:1203–1213.

Orhan IE et al 2012. Antimicrobial and antiviral effects of essential oils from selected Umbelliferae and Labiatae plants and individual essential oil components. Turkish Journal of Biology; 36(3):239–246.

Ostad SN et al 2001. The effect of fennel essential oil on uterine contraction as a model for dysmenorrhea, pharmacology and toxicology study. J Ethnopharmacol; 76(3):299–304.

Ozbek H et al 2003. Hepatoprotective effect of *Foeniculum vulgare* essential oil. Fitoterapia; 74(3):317–319.

Pazoki H et al 2016. Comparing the effects of aerobic exercise and Foeniculum vulgare on pre-menstrual syndrome. Middle East Fertil Soc J. 2016; 21:61–64.

Pourabbas S et al 2001. Study of the anxiolytic effects of fennel and possible roles of both gaba-ergic system and estrogen receptors in these effects in adult female rat. Physiol Pharmacol; 15:134–143.

Shakkant B et al 2014. Foeniculum vulgare Mill: A Review of its botany, phytochemistry, pharmacology, contemporary application and toxicology. Biomed Res Int. 842674. Published online doi: 10.1155/2014/842674.

Yaralizadeh M et al 2016. Effect of *Foeniculum vulgare* (fennel) vaginal cream on vaginal atrophy in postmenopausal women: a double-blind randomized placebo-controlled trial. Maturitas; 84:75–80.

Chapter 8 Fumitory *Fumaria officinalis*
Drawing of Fumitory: Step, Edward Wayside and woodland blossoms (Pl 8) (8746623835).jpg.

Chapter 9 Iris *Iris germanica*
Drawing of iris by François Rozier, Cours d'agriculture, tome 5, planche 29.

Chapter 10 Ivy *Hedera helix*
Drawing of ivy (Header helix) fruiting branch: Anonymous

Al-Snafi AE 2018. Pharmacological and therapeutic activities of *Hedera helix*- A review. IOSR J Pharm 8(5) Version. I; 41–53.

Amara-Mokrane YA et al 1996. Protective effects of alfa-hederin, chlorophyllin and ascorbic acid towards the induction of micronuclei by doxorubicin in cultured human lymphocytes. Mutagenesis; 11:161–7.

Büechi S et al 2005. Open trial to assess aspects of safety and efficacy of a combined herbal cough syrup with ivy and thyme. Forsch Komplementarmed Klass Naturheilkd; 12(6): 328–332. Cwientzek U et al 2011. Acute bronchitis therapy with ivy leaves extracts in a two-arm study. A double-blind, randomised study vs. another ivy leaves extract. Phytomed; 18(13):1105–1109. Chichiricco G et al 1980. Phytotherapy in the subequana valley, Abruzzo, central Italy. J Ethnopharmacol; 2: 247–257.

Elias R et al 1990. Antimutagenic activity of some saponins isolated from **Calendula** *officinalis* L., *C. arvensis* L. and *Hedera helix* L. Mutagenesis; 5(4):327–331.

European Medicines Agency 2011, Committee on Herbal Medicinal Products; Assessment report on *Hedera helix* L., folium; European Medicines Agency, London.

European Pharmacopoeia. 7th ed. Monograph. 01/2008:2148.

Fazio S et al 2009. Tolerance, safety and efficacy of *Hedera helix* extract in inflammatory bronchial diseases under clinical practice conditions: a prospective, open, multicentre postmarketing study in 9657 patients. Phytomed; 16(1):17–24.

Grieves M 1931. A Modern Herbal.

Hocaoglu AB et al 2012. Effect of *Hedera helix* on lung histopathology in chronic asthma. Iran. J

Hofmann D et al 2003. Efficacy of dry extract of ivy leaves in children with bronchial asthma-a review of randomized controlled trials. Phytomedicine; 10(2–3): 213–220.

Kemmerich B et al 2006. Efficacy and tolerability of a fluid extract combination of thyme herb and ivy leaves and matched placebo in adults suffering from acute bronchitis with productive cough: A prospective, double-blind, placebo- controlled clinical trial. Arzneim; 56(9): 652–660.

Medeiros JR et al 2002. Bioactive components of *Hedera helix*. Arquipélago, Life and Marine Sciences; 19A: 27–32.

Mendel M et al 2011. The effect of the whole extract of common ivy (*Hedera helix*) leaves and selected active substances on the motoric activity of rat isolated stomach strips. J Ethnopharmacol; 134(3): 796–802.

Mendel M et al 2013. Participation of extracellular calcium in α-hederin-induced contractions of rat isolated stomach strips. J Ethnopharmacol; 146(1):423–426.

Mulkijanyan K et al 2013. Ivy water extracts as gastric ulcer preventive agents. Georgian Med News; (224):63–66. Rai A 2013. The Anti-inflammatory and anti-arthritic properties of ethanol extract of *Hedera helix*. Indian J Pharm Sci; 75(1):99–102.

Rashed KNZ 2013. Antioxidant activity of *Hedera helix* L. extracts and the main phytoconstituents. Int J of Allied Med Sci and Clin Res; 1(2): 62–64.

Rauf A et al 2014. Analgesic and antioxidant activity of crude extracts and isolated fractions of aerial parts of *Hedera helix* L. JSM Chem; 2(2): 1012.

Schmidt M, Thomsen M and Schmidt U. Suitability of ivy extract for the treatment of paediatric cough. Phytother Res 2012; 26(12):1942–1947.

Schulte-Michels J et al 2016. Ivy leaves dry extract EA 575® decreases LPS-induced IL-6 release from murine macrophages. Pharmazie; 71(3):158–161.

Sieben A et al 2009. Alpha-hederin, but not hederacoside C and hederagenin from *Hedera helix*, affects the binding behaviour, dynamics, and regulation of beta 2-adrenergic receptors. Biochem; 48(15):3477–3482.

Trute A et al 1997. *In vitro* antispasmodic compounds of the dry extract obtained from Hedera helix. Planta Med; 63(2): 125–129.

Wolf A et al 2011. Pre-treatment with α-hederin increases beta-adrenoceptor mediated relaxation of airway smooth muscle. Phytomed; 18(2–3): 214–218.

Chapter 11 Juniper *Juniperus communis*
Drawing of Juniper from the Wellcome collection M0005902.jpg.

Chapter 12 Laurel or *Bay Laurus nobilis*
Drawing by the author.

Chapter 13 Lemon *Citrus limon*
Drawing of lemon tree (Citrus limon): branch with fruit and flowers. Charcoal drawing by E. Shepperd, 1894. Wellcome V0044542.jpg.

Aboelhadid SM et al 2016. *In vitro* and in vivo effect of *Citrus limon* essential oil against sarcoptic mange in rabbits. Parasitol Res; 115: 3013–3020.

Bhavsar SK et al 2007. Investigation into hepato-protective activity of *Citrus limon*. Pharm. Biol; 45: 303–311.

European Directorate for the Quality of Medicines. European Pharmacopoeia 9.2, Lemon Oil. Strasburg, Germany: 2017.

Hamdan D et al 2013. Chemical composition of the essential oils of variegated pink-fleshed lemon (*Citrus* x *limon* L. Burm. f.) and their anti-inflammatory and antimicrobial activities. Zeitschrift fur Naturforsch. -Sect. C J. Biosci; 68C: 275–284.

Lima NGPB et al 2013. Anxiolytic-like activity and GC-MS analysis of (R)-(+)-limonene fragrance, a natural compound found in foods and plants. Pharmacol Biochem Behav; 103:450–454.

McGee H 2004. McGee on food and cooking: an encyclopaedia of kitchen science, history and culture. Hodder and Stoughton ISBN 0340831499.

Millet F 2014. Huiles essentielles et essence de citronnier (*Citrus limon* (L.) Burm. f.) Phytotherapie; 12: 89–97.

Ministry of Health and Family Welfare. The Ayurvedic Pharmacopoeia of India (IV) Government of India; New Delhi, India: 2017. *Citrus limon* (Lilnn) Burm.

Mohanapriya M et al 2013. Health and medicinal properties of lemon (*Citrus limonum*) Int J Ayurvedic Herb Med; 1: 1095–1100.

Morton JF 1987. Lemon in Fruits of Warm Climates. Purdue University. 160–168.

Murali R and Saravanan R 2012. Antidiabetic effect of d-limonene, a monoterpene in streptozotocin-induced diabetic rats. Biomed. Prev. Nutr; 2:269–275.

Otang WM and Afolayan AJ 2016. Antimicrobial and antioxidant efficacy of *Citrus limon* L. peel extracts used for skin diseases by Xhosa tribe of Amathole District, Eastern Cape, South Africa. S. Afr. J. Bot; 102:46–49.

Parhiz H et al 2015. Antioxidant and anti-inflammatory properties of the citrus flavonoids hesperidin and hesperein:

An updated review of their molecular mechanisms and experimental models. Phyther Res 29:323–331.

Raimondo S et al 2015. *Citrus limon*-derived nanovesicles inhibit cancer cell proliferation and suppress CML xenograft growth by inducing TRAIL-mediated cell death. Oncotarget; 6:19514–19527.

Tsujiyama I et al 2013. Anti-histamine release and anti-inflammatory activities of aqueous extracts of citrus fruits peels. Orient Pharm Exp Med; 13: 175–180.

The United States Pharmacopeial Convention. United States Pharmacopoeia. National Formulary. Rockville, MD, USA: 2009.

Chapter 14 Myrtle *Myrtus communis*

Drawing of myrtle by Prof. Dr. Otto Wilhelm Thomé *Flora von Deutschland, Österreich und der Schweiz* 1885, Gera, Germany. Permission granted to use under GFDL by Kurt Stueber.

Chapter 15 Mustard *Brassica nigra*

Drawing of mustard by the author.

Bhattacharya A et al 2010. Allyl isothiocyanate-rich mustard seed powder inhibits bladder cancer growth and muscle invasion. Carcinogenesis 12: 2105–2110.

Chou T-C 2008. Preclinical versus clinical drug combination studies. Leuk Lymphoma; 49: 2059–2080.

John P and Aravindakshan CM 2012. Hypolipidemic effect of *Brassica juncea* (mustard) in alloxan induced diabetic rats. JIVA; 10(2): 13–16.

Kim HY et al 2003. *In vitro* and *in vivo* antioxidant effects of mustard leaf (*Brassica juncea*). Phyto Res. 2003;17(5): 465–471.

Mejía-Garibay B, et al 2015. Composition, diffusion, and anti-fungal activity of black mustard (*Brassica nigra*) essential oil when applied by direct addition or vapour contact. J Food Prot; 78(4): 843–848.

Nauman S and Mohammad I 2015. Role of khardal (*Brassica nigra*) in non-communicable diseases: an overview. Int J Drug Dev Res; 7(1): 137–144.

Rajamurugan R et al 2012. *Brassica nigra* plays a remedy role in hepatic and renal damage. Pharm Biol; 50(12): 1488–1497.

Thakur AK et al 2013. Beneficial effects of *Brassica juncea* on cognitive function in rats. Pharm Biol; 51(10): 1304–1310.

Tripathi K et al. 2015 Allyl isothiocyanate induces replication-associated DNA damage response in NSCLC cells and sensitizes to ionizing radiation. Oncotarget, 6: 5237–5252.

Tseng E et al 2002. Effect of organic isothiocyanates on the P-glycoprotein- and MRP1-mediated transport of daunomycin and vinblastine. Pharm Res; 19 (10): 1509–1515.

Xie Q et al 2014. Sensitization of cancer cells to radiation by selenadiazole derivatives by regulation of ROS-mediated DNA damage and ERK and AKT pathways. Biochem Biophys Res Commun; 449: 88–93.

Yadav SP et al 2004. *Brassica juncea* (rai) significantly prevented the development of insulin resistance in rats fed fructose-enriched diet. J Ethnopharmacol; 93 (1): 113–116.

Chapter 16 Olive *Olea europea*

Al-Azzawie HF and Alhamdani MS 2006. Hypoglycemic and antioxidant effect of oleuropein in alloxan-diabetic rabbits. Life Sci 78: 1371–1377.

Al-Qarawi AA et al 2002. Effect of freeze dried extract of *Olea europaea* on the pituitary-thyroid axis in rats. Phytotherapy Res 16: 286–287.

Apollodorus The Library. Trans JG Frazer 1963–1967. Loeb Classical library Cabridge MA, Harvard Uni Press.

Benavent-Garcia O et al 2000. Antioxidant activity of phenolics extracted from *Olea europaea* L. Leaves. Food chem 68: 457–462.

Bennani-Kabchi N et al 1999. Effects of *Olea europea var. oleaster* leaves in hyper-cholesterolemic insulin-resistant sand rats. Therapie 54 (6): 717–23.

Bisignano G et al 1999. On the *in-vitro* anti-microbial activity of oleuropein and hydroxytyrosol. J Pharm Pharmacol 51 (8): 971–974.

Briante R et al 2002. *Olea europaea* L. Leaf extract and derivatives: antioxidant properties. J Agric Food Chem 50: 4934–4940.

Capretti G and Bonaconza E 1949. Effect of infusion of decoctions of olive leaves (*Olea europaea*) on some physical constants of blood (viscosity and surface tension) and on some. Giorn Clin Med.

Caturla N 2005. Differential effects of oleuropein, a biophenol from *Olea europaea*, on anionic and zwiterionic phospholipid model membranes. Chem Phys Lipids 137: 2–17.

Chimi H et al 1995. Inhibition of iron toxicity in rat hepatocyte culture by natural phenolic compounds. Tox *in vitro* 9: 695–702.

Cruess WV 1915–1965 Papers.

De Bock M et al 2013. Olive (*Olea europaea* L.) leaf polyphenols improve insulin sensitivity in middle-aged overweight men: a randomised placebo-controlled, crossover trial. PloS one 8 (3), e57622.

De Nino L et al 2005. Absolute method for the assay of oleuropein in olive oils by atmospheric pressure chemical ionisation tandem mass spectrometry. Anal Chem 77: 5961–5964.

Gonzalez M et al 1992. Hypoglycemic activity of olive leaf. Planta Med 58: 513–515.

Gorini F 2023. Olive oil times.

Hanbury D 1874. Pharmacographia Macmillan.

Hanbury D 1841. Trans Pharmaceut Soc. 1. London: J and A Churchill.

Hansen K et al 1996. Isolation of an angiotensin converting enzyme (ACE) inhibitor from *Olea europaea* and *Olea lacea*. Phytomedicine 2: 319–325.

Heinze JE et al 1975. Specificity of the anti-viral agent calcium elenolate. Anti-microbial Agents Chemother 8 (4): 421–5.

Khan Y 2007. *Olea europaea*: A Phyto-Pharmacological Review. Pharmacog Rev 1 (1).

Kushi LH et al 1995. Health implications of Mediterranean diets in light of contemporary knowledge. Meat, wine, fats and oils. Am J Clin Nutr 61: 1416S–1427S.

Perrinjaquet-Moccetti T 2008. Food supplementation with an olive (*Olea europaea* L.) leaf extract reduces blood pressure in borderline hypertensive monozygotic twins. Phytother Res 22 (9): 1239–1242.

Petroni A et al 1995. Inhibition of platelet aggregation and eicosanoid production by phenolic components of olive oil. Thromb Res 78 (2): 151–160.

Petkov V and Manolov P 1972. Pharmacological analysis of the iridoid oleuropein. Drug Res 22 (9): 1476–86.

Pieroni A et al 1996. *In vitro* anti-complementary activity of flavonoids from olive (*Olea europaea* L) leaves. Pharmazie 51 (10): 765–768.

Renis HE 1970. *In vitro* anti-viral activity of calcium elenolate. Anti-microbial Agents Chemother 167–72.

Shesh A 2005. The Herbs of Avurveda 3: 820.

Soret MC 1969. Anti-viral activity of calcium elenolate on parainfluenza infection of hamsters. Anti-microbial Agents and Chemother 9: 160–66.

Susalit E 2011. Olive (Olea europaea) leaf extract effective in patients with stage-1 hypertension: Comparison with Captopril. Phytomed 18 (4): 251–258.

Susalit E 2011. Olive (Olea europaea) leaf extract effective in patients with stage-1 hypertension: Comparison with Captopril. Phytomed 18 (4): 251–258.

Visioli F et al 1994. Oleuropein protects low density lipoprotein from oxidation. Life Sci 55: 71.

Visioli F et al 2002. Antioxidant and other biological activities of phenols from olives and olive oil. Med Res Rev 22: 65–75.

Weinstein J 2012. Olive leaf extract as a hypoglycaemic agent in both human diabetic subjects and in rats. J Med Food 15 (7)

Zarzuelo A et al 1991. Vasodilator effect of olive leaf. Planta Med. 57 (5): 417–9.

Zaslaver M et al 2005. Natural compounds derived from foods modulate nitric oxide production and oxidative status in epithelial lung cells. J Agric Food Chem., 53: 9934–9939.

Chapter 17 Orpine *Sedum telephium* or *Hylotelephium telephium*

Drawing by the author.

Balatri S 2013. Piante Medicinali, 12: 3–5.

Biagi M et al 2013. Piante Medicinali, 12: 6–9.

Bonina F et al 2000. J Pharm Pharmacol.

Guarrera PM 2006. Usi e Tradizioni della Flora Italiana. Medicina popolare ed etnobotanica. Aracne, Roma.

Huang D et al 2010. Antitumour activity of the aqueous extract from *Sedum sarmentosum* Bunge in vitro. J Cancer Biother Radiopharm: 25(1): 81–88.

Ligaa U 1996. Medicinal plants of Mongolia used in Mongolian traditional medicine. Seoul, Korea, 339–340.

Matsuda H et al 2001. Dimeric sesquiterpene thio-alkaloids with potent immunosuppressive activity from the rhizome of *Nuphar pumilum*: structural requirements of nuphar alkaloids for immunosuppressive activity. Bioorg Med Chem; 9(4): 1031–1035.

Silva-Torres R et al 2003. Spermicidal activity of the crude ethanol extract of *Sedum praealtum* in mice. J Ethnopharmacol: 85(1): 15–17.

Vitalini S et al 2015. J. Ethnopharmacol; 173: 435.

Qin F and Sun HX 2008. Immunosuppressive activity of the ethanol extract of *Sedum sarmentosum* and its fractions on specific antibody and cellular responses to ovalbumin in mice. Chemistry and Biodiversity 5(12): 2699–2709.

Chapter 18 Rhubarb *Rheum rhabarbarum*

Brkanac SR et al 1015. Toxicity and antioxidant capacity of *Frangula alnus* Mill. bark and its active component emodin. Regul Toxicol Pharmacol; 73: 923–929.

Chen X et al 2015. Physcion induces mitochondria-driven apoptosis in colorectal cancer cells via down-regulating EMMPRIN. Eur J Pharmacol; 764: 124–133.

Chen YK et al 2016. Emodin alleviates jejunum injury in rats with sepsis by inhibiting inflammation response. Biomed Pharmacother; 84: 1001–1007.

Cui Y et al 2016. Involvement of PI3K/Akt, ERK and p38 signaling pathways in emodin-mediated extrinsic and intrinsic human hepatoblastoma cell apoptosis. Food Chem Toxicol; 92: 26–37.

Dong GZ et al 2015. Stilbenoids from *Rheum undulatum* protect hepatocytes against oxidative stress through AMPK activation. Phytother Res 29:1605–1609.

Fu XS et al 2011. Progress in research of chemical constituents and pharmacological actions of Rhubarb. Chin J New Drugs; 20: 1534–1538.

Ji YS 2000. Pharmacology and application of active ingredients of Traditional Chinese Medicine. Beijing: People's Medical Publishing House; 95–117.

Jiao D and Du SJ 2000. *Study on rhubarb.* Shanghai: Shanghai Science and Technology Press; pp. 273–307.

Kalpana D et al 2012. GC-MS analysis and evaluation of antimicrobial, free radical scavenging and *in vitro* cytotoxic activities of the methanolic extract of *Rheum undulatum*. Sci Adv Mater 4:1238–1246.

Kosikowska U et al 2010. Antimicrobial activity and total content of polyphenols of *Rheum* L. species growing in Poland. Cent Eur J Biol 5(6):814–820.

Li HL et al 2005. Isorhapontigenin, a new resveratrol analog, attenuates cardiac hypertrophy via blocking signalling transduction pathways. Free Radic Biol Med; 38: 243–257.

Li L et al 2016. The antibacterial activity and action mechanism of emodin from *Polygonum cuspidatum* against *Haemophilus parasuis* in vitro. Microbiol Res; 186–187: 139–145.

Liu HF and Zhang CY 2016. Comprehensive nursing rhubarb compound enema decoction high colon dialysis treatment for diabetic nephropathy phase IV and V clinical observation. Hu Li Tian Di; 1: 184–186.

Lu L et al 2014. Rhubarb root and rhizome-based Chinese herbal prescriptions for acute ischemic stroke: a systematic review and meta-analysis. Complement Ther Med; 22: 1060–1070.

McDougall GJ et al 2010. Effect of different cooking regimes on rhubarb polyphenols. Food Chem 119:758–764.

Sui F et al 2012. Comparison of the actions on blood stasis of rhubarb with different prepared methods. Chin Med Pharmaco Clinic; 6: 90–93.

Su J et al 2011. Influence of rhein intervention on the expression of HGF and BMP7 in renal tissue of rats with chronical allograft nephropathy. Chin J Clin Pharmacol; 16: 1114–1120.

Sun BQ and Zhu GB 2017. Clinical observation on treatment of rhubarb and mirabilite on severe acute pancreatitis. J Emerg Tradit Chin Med; 23: 1155–1156.

Tabolacci C et al 2015. Aloe-emodin exerts a potent anticancer and immunomodulatory activity on BRAF-mutated human melanoma cells. Eur J Pharmacol; 762: 283–292.

Tan ZH et al 2004. Effects of rhein on the function of human mesangial cells in high glucose environment. Acta Pharm Sin; 39: 881–886.

Tong Y and Jin Z 2015. Research progress of pharmacological effect of physcion. Chin Arch Tradit Chin Med; 33: 938–940.

Wang RQ 2007. Clinical observation of the treatment of micron rhubarb charcoal in peptic ulcer bleeding and the mechanism of platelet system. Master, Hubei College of Traditional Chinese Medicine, Hubei, China.

Wang L and Pan S 2015. Adjuvant treatment with crude rhubarb for patients with acute organophosphorus pesticide poisoning: a meta-analysis of randomized controlled trials. Complement Ther Med; 23: 794–801.

Wang H et al 2012. *Rheum officinale* (a Traditional Chinese Medicine) for chronic kidney disease. Cochrane Database Syst Rev. 7.

Wang LL et al 2015 The influence of free anthraquinone of rhubarb in severe acute pancreatitis induced kidney injury. Chin Med Pharmaco Clin; 31: 31–34.

Wang SZ 2015. Forty cases with upper gastrointestinal hemorrhage treated with oral administration of raw dahuang powder. Henan Trad Chin Med; 35: 2798–2799.

Wang YM et al 2008. Effects of rhubarb polysaccharide on blood glucose, blood lipids, hepatic lipase activity in rats with diabetic atherosclerosis. Mod Med J Chin; 10: 6–9.

Wang ZW et al 2015. Effects of rhubarbs from different regions on blood lipid and antioxidation of hyperlipidemia rats. Chin J Appl Physiol; 31: 278–281.

Xie Y et al 1016. Research progress in rhubarb polysaccharides. Chin J New Drugs; 19: 755–758.

Xiong ZH 2012. The study of intervention effect and molecular mechanism of rhubarb used in diabetic nephropathy. Doctor, Guangzhou University of Chinese Medicine. Guangzhou, China.

Zeng LN et al 2013. The protective and toxic effects of rhubarb tannins and anthraquinones in treating hexavalent chromium-injured rats: the Yin/Yang actions of rhubarb. J Hazard Mater; 246–247: 1–9.

Zhang Y et al 2013. Protective effect of rhubarb free anthraquinone on intestinal barrier injury in beagle dogs induced by severe acute pancreatitis. Chin J Exp Tradit Med Form; 19: 172–176.

Zhao YM et al 2016. Neuroprotective effects of chrysophanol against inflammation in middle cerebral artery occlusion in mice. Neurosci Lett; 630: 16–22.

Zhong HY et al 2006. Effect of tannin contained in Radix et Rhizoma Rhei and Radix Polygoni Multiflori on small intestinal propulsion. Lishizhen Med Mater Med Res; 17: 2478–2479.

Zhou Y et al 2016. Add-on effect of crude rhubarb to somatostatin for acute pancreatitis: a meta-analysis of randomized controlled trials. J Ethnopharmacol; 194: 495–505.

Zhu W and Wang XM 2005. Progress in study on mechanisms of rhubarb in treating chronic renal failure. Chin J Integr Trad West Med; 25: 471–475.

Chapter 19 Rose *Rosa spp*

Pozzi G 2018. La Parola Dipinta. Adelphi.

Chapter 20 Sage *Salvia officinalis*

Drawing by the author.

Chapter 22 Sorrel *Rumex acetosa*

Drawing by Reichenbach, Heinrich Gottlieb Ludwig.

Alzoreky N and Nakahara K 2001. Anti-oxidant activity of some edible Yemeni plants evaluated by Ferrymyoglobin ABTS+assay. Food Sci Technol Res 7: 141–144.

Bae J-Y et al 2012. A comparison between water and ethanol extracts of *Rumex acetosa* for protective effects on gastric ulcers in mice. Biomol Ther. 20: 425–430.

Beckert S and Hensel A, 2013. Proteinase-inhibiting activity of an extract of *Rumex acetosa* L. against virulence factors of *Porphyromonas gingivalis*. Planta Med; 79.

Brinker F J 1998. Herb Contraindications and Drug Interactions. (2nd ed), Eclectic Medical Publications, Sandy, OR.

Gescher K et al., 2011 Oligomeric proanthocyanidins from Rumex acetosa L. inhibit the attachment of herpes simplex virus type-1Antiviral Res., 89 (2011), pp. 9–18.

Jund R et al 2012. Clinical efficacy of a dry extract of five herbal drugs in acute viral rhino-sinusitis Rhinology, 50; 417–426.

Mimica-Dukić N 2016. Native plants in Serbia as a source of new anti-inflammatory agents - the case of *Polygonaceae* Family. XV Optima Meeting June 6–11, Montpellier.

Schmuch J et al 2015. Extract from *Rumex acetosa* L. for prophylaxis of periodontitis: inhibition of bacterial *in vitro* adhesion and of *gingipains* of *Porphyromonas gingivalis* by epicatechin-3-O-(4β → 8)-epicatechin-3-O-gallate (procyanidin-B2-Digallate.) PLoS One 10. 1371 J pone. 0120130.

Part 3 Exotic Healing Plants Used in Renaissance Florence

Chapter 1 Balm of Gilead *Commiphora gileadensis*

Drawing by Luigi Balugani: B1977,14,8904-Yale Centre for British Art.jpg.

Abdul-Ghani AS and Amin R 1997. Effect of aqueous extract of *Commiphora opobalsamum* on blood pressure and heart rate in rats. J Ethnopharmacological 57: 219–222.

Alhazmi A 2022. Antibacterial effects of *Commiphora gileadensis* methanol extract on wound healing molecules. Molecules 21; 27(10): 3320.

al-Howiriny TA et al 2004. Studies on the pharmacological activities of an ethanol extract of Balsean, *Commiphora opobalsamum*. Pak J Biol Sci 7; 1933–1936.

al-Howiriny T et al 2005. Effect of *Commiphora opobalsamum* (L.) Engl. (Balessan) on experimental gastric ulcers and secretion in rats. J Ethnopharmacol 98: 287–294.

Al-Mahbashi HM 2015. Evaluation of acute toxicity and antimicrobial effects of the bark extract of Bisham (*Commiphora gileadensis* L.) J Chem and Pharm Res. 7(6): 810–814.

Al-sieni AI 2014. The antibacterial activity of traditionally used *Salvadora Persia* L (miswak) and *Commiphora gileadensis* (palsam) in Saudi Arabia. Air J Tradit Complement Altern Med: AJTCAM/FRI NETW ETHNOMED 11; 23–27.

Anwar D'a 2016. Therapeutic and preventive effects of *Commiphora gileadensis* against diethylnitrosamine-induced hepatic injury in albino rats. African Journal of Pharmacy and Pharmacology 10(16). 356–363.

Chan et al 2012. Mitosis-targeted anti-cancer therapies: where they stand. Cell Death Dis 3: 411.

Gilboa-Garber and Zohar A 2010. Medicinal properties of *Commiphora gileadensis*. African J Pharm and Pharmacol 4(8); 516–520.

Haddad A et al 2020. The antioxidant and antidiabetic activity of the Arabian balsam tree *Commiphora gileadensis* in hyperlipidaemic male rats. J Taibah Uni Sci 14, 1.

Hepper NF and Taylor JE 2004. Date palms and opobalsam in the Madaba Mosaic map. Palestine Explor Q 136; 35–44

Lev E 2002. "Reconstructed Materia Medica of the Medieval and Ottoman al-Sham," J Ethnopharmacol, 80(2–3): 167–179.

Shen T et al 2007. Secondary metabolites from *Commiphora opobalsamum* and their anti proliferative effect on human prostate cancer cells. Phytochem 68: 1331–1337.

Wineman E 2015. *Commiphora gileadensis* sap extract induces cell cycle-dependent death in immortalised keratinocytes and human dermoid carcinoma cells. J Herbal Med 5 (4): 199–206.

Zohary M 1982. Plants of the Bible: A complete handbook to all the plants with 200 full colour plates taken in the natural habitat. Cambridge University Press, London UK.

Chapter 2 Camphor Tree *Cinnamomum camphora*

Camphor Tree Chromolithograph, c. 1887, after W. Müller.

Ansari MA and Razdan RK 1995. Relative efficacy of various oils in repelling mosquitoes. Indian J. Malariol; 32: 104–111.

Brent H et al 1990. Conditioning: A New Approach to Immunotherapy. American Association for Cancer Research; 50: 4295–299.

Burrow A et al 1983. The effects of camphor, eucalyptus and menthol vapour on nasal resistance to airflow and nasal sensation. Acta Otolaryngol 96: 157–161.

Chen-Lung H et al 2009. Essential Oil Compositions and Bioactivities of the Various Parts of *Cinnamomum camphora* Sieb.Var. Linaloolifera Fujuta; 31(2): 77–96.

Edris AE 2007. Pharmaceutical and Therapeutic Potentials of Essential Oils and Their Individual Volatile Constituents: A Review; 308–23.

Frizzo CD et al 2000. Essential Oils of Camphor Tree (*Cinnamomum Camphora* Nees & Eberm) Cultivated in Southern Brazil. Brazilian Archives of Biology and Technology; 43(3).

Ghanta VK et al 1990. Conditioning: a new approach to immunotherapy. Cancer Res 50(14); 4295–9.

Hamidpour R et al 2012. Camphor (*Cinnamomum camphora*) a traditional remedy with the history of treating several diseases. IJCRI.

Kaegi E 1998. Unconventional Therapies for Cancer: 714-X. Canadian Medical Association Journal 1998, 158(12):1621–624.

Kumar M and Youshinori A 2003. Single-wall and Multi- wall Carbon Nanotubes from Camphor-A Botanical Hydrocarbon. Diamond and Related Materials; 12: 1845–850.

Kumar M and Youshinori A 2007. Carbon Nanotubes from Camphor: An Environment-Friendly Nanotechnology. Journal of Physics Conferences Series; 61: 643–46.

Lin CT et al 2007. Bioactivity Investigation of Lauraceae Trees Grown in Taiwan. Pharmaceutical Biology; 45(8): 638–44.

Ling J and Liu WY 1996. Cytotoxicity of Two New Ribosome-Inactivating Proteins, Cinnamomin and Camphorin, to Carcinoma Cells. Cell Biochem Funct; 14(3): 157–61.

Liu R-S et al 2002. Cinnamomin, A Type II Ribosome-Inactivating Protein, Is A Storage Protein in the Seed of the Camphor Tree (*Cinnamomum Camphora*). Biochemical Society Journal; 362: 659–63.

Salman AS et al 2012. Protective Effect of *Cinnamomum Camphora* Leaves Extract against Atrazine Induced Genotoxicity and Biochemical Effect on Mice. Journal of American Science; 8(1): 190–96.

Sydney S et al 1978. Camphor: Who Needs It? American Academy of Pediatrics; 62(3): 404–06.

Weiss L et al 2011. Herbal Flavonoids Inhibit the Development of Autoimmune Diabetes in NOD Mice: Proposed Mechanisms of Action in the Example of PADMA 28. Alternative Medicine Studies. (e1):1–6.

Zuccarini P 2009. Camphor: Risks and Benefits of a Widely Used Natural Product. J. Appl. Sci. Environ. Manage;13(2):69–74.

Chapter 3 Cinnamon *Cinnamomum verum*

Picture of cinnamon from popular bible encyclopedia of Archimandrite Nicephorus (1892).

Abascal K and Yarnell E 2010. The medicinal uses of cinnamon. Integrative Med; 9(1): 28–32.

Brahmachari S et al 2009. Sodium benzoate, a metabolite of cinnamon and a food additive, reduces microglial and astroglial inflammatory responses. J Immunol. 183, (9); 5917–5927.

Chang ST et al 2001. Antibacterial activity of leaf essential oils and their constituents from *Cinnamomum osmophloeum.* J Ethnopharmacol, 77(1); 123–127.

Cheng SS et al 2004. Chemical composition and mosquito larvicidal activity of essential oils from leaves of different *Cinnamomum osmophloeum* provenances," J Agric Food Chem 52(14); 4395–4400.

Frydman-Marom A et al 2011. Orally administrated cinnamon extract reduces β-amyloid oligomerization and corrects cognitive impairment in Alzheimer's disease animal models. PLoS ONE. 6(1); Article ID e16564.

Harada M and Yano S 1975. Pharmacological studies on Chinese cinnamon. II. Effects of cinnamaldehyde on the cardiovascular and digestive systems. Chem and Pharm Bull. 23(5): 941–947.

Hossein N et al 2013. Effect of *Cinnamon sylanicum* essence and distillate on the clotting time. J Med Plants Res 7 (19); 1339–1343.

Hwa JS et al 2012. 2-Methoxycinnamaldehyde from *Cinnamomum cassia* reduces rat myocardial ischemia and reperfusion injury *in vivo* due to HO-1 induction. J Ethnopharmacol. 139(2): 605–615.

Kim SH et al 2006. Anti-diabetic effect of cinnamon extract on blood glucose in db/db mice," J Ethnopharmacol, 104(1–2); 119–123.

Lee EJ et al 2009. Therapeutic window for cinnamophilin following oxygen-glucose deprivation and transient focal cerebral ischemia. Experimental Neurology. 217(1); 74–83.

Lee HS et al 2002. Suppression effect of *Cinnamomum cassia* bark-derived component on nitric oxide synthase. J Agric Food Chem. 50 (26) 7700–7703.

Lin J et al 1999. Preliminary screening of some traditional Zulu medicinal plants for anti-inflammatory and anti-microbial activities," J Ethnopharmacol. 68(1–3); 267–274.

Lu J et al 2009. Novel angiogenesis inhibitory activity in cinnamon extract blocks VEGFR2 kinase and downstream signaling," Carcinogenesis 31(3); 481–488.

Mancini-Filho J et al 1998. Antioxidant activity of cinnamon (*Cinnamomum zeylanicum*, breyne) extracts," Bollettino Chimico Farmaceutico, 137(11); 443–447.

Mansoure R 2014. The Effect of Tea-Cinnamon and *Melissa officinalis* L. Aqueous Extraction, on Neuropsychology Distress, Biochemical and Oxidative Stress Biomarkers in Glass Production Workers. Health 06(19). Article ID:51337, 9 pages.

Okawa M et al 2001. DPPH (1,1-diphenyl-2-Picrylhydrazyl) radical scavenging activity of flavonoids obtained from some medicinal plants. Biolog Pharm Bull, 24(10); 1202–1205.

Park I-K et al 2005. Nematicidal activity of plant essential oils and components from garlic (*Allium sativum*) and cinnamon (*Cinnamomum verum*) oils against the pine wood nematode (Bursaphelenchus xylophilus)," Nematology, vol. 7, no. 5, pp. 767–774.

Sangal A 2011. "Role of cinnamon as beneficial anti-diabetic food adjunct: a review," Advances in Applied Science Research, vol. 2, no. 4, pp. 440–450, 2011.

Shobana S and Akhilender Naidu K 2000. Antioxidant activity of selected Indian spices. Prostaglandins Leukotrienes and Essential Fatty Acids 62(2); 107–110.

Singletary K 2019. Cinnamon Update of Potential Health Benefits. Nutrition Today. 1/2; 54(1); 42–52.

Song F et al 2013. Protective effects of cinnamic acid and cinnamic aldehyde on isoproterenol-induced acute myocardial ischemia in rats. J Ethnopharmacol. 150(1):125–130.

Tung Y-T et al 2008. Anti-inflammation activities of essential oil and its constituents from indigenous cinnamon (*Cinnamomum osmophloeum*) twigs. Bioresource Tech, 99(9); 3908–3913.

Yu SM et al 1994. Cinnamophilin, a novel thromboxane A2 receptor antagonist, isolated from *Cinnamomum philippinense.* European J Pharmacol. 256(1); 85–91.

Wang S-Y et al 2005. Antifungal activities of essential oils and their constituents from indigenous cinnamon (*Cinnamomum osmophloeum*) leaves against wood decay fungi," Bioresource Technol, 96(7); 813–818.

Chapter 4 Dragon's Blood Tree *Dracaena draco*

Drawing of Dragon's blood tree by Caroli Clusii in: atrebat Rariorum alioquot stirpium per Hispanias observatarum historia (Page 12) HHL 7813824.jpg.

Ansari MJ 2016. Antimicrobial activity of Dracaena cinnabar resin from Soqotra Island on multi drug resistant human pathogens. African J Trad Comp Alternat Med 13(1).

Camarda L et al 2011. Ch. 11. New York, NY, USA: Nova Science Publishers Inc; In Resin Composites: Properties, Production and Applications; 353–74.

Di Stefano et al 2014. Phytochemical and anti-staphylococcal biofilm assessment of *Dracaena draco* L. Spp. *draco* resin. Pharmacogn Mag 10(suppl 2); S434-S440.

González AG et al 2003. Steroidal saponins from the bark of *Dracaena draco* and their cytotoxic activities. J Nat Prod. 66:793–8.

Gupta D et al 2008. Dragon's blood: Botany, chemistry and therapeutic uses. J Ethnopharmacol. 115:361–80.

Gupta D & Gupta RK 2011. Bioprotective properties of Dragon's blood resin: *In vitro* evaluation of antioxidant activity and antimicrobial activity. 11(13).

Israa AI et al 2018. Bioactivities, characterisation and therapeutic uses of *Dracaena cinnabari*. Int J Pharm Qual Assur 9; 11–14.

Melo MJ et al 2007. Identification of 7,4-Dihydroxy-5-methoxyflavylium in "Dragon's Blood": To be or not to be an anthocyanin. Chemistry; 13:1417–22.

Milburn M 1984. Dragon's Blood in East and West Africa, Arabia and the Canary Islands. Africa. 39:486–93.

Shu J et al 2015. *Sanguis Draconis* (*Daemonorops draco*) A Case Report of Treating a Chronic Pressure Ulcer With Tunneling. Holistic Nursing Practice. 29 (1): 48–52.

Silva BM 2011. *Dracaena draco* L. fruit: Phytochemical and antioxidant activity assessment. Food Res Int 44 (7); 2182–2189.

Chapter 5 Lemon Grass *Cymbopogon citratus*

Picture of lemongrass: encyclopaedia of the Plant_Kingdom. pic136.jpg.

Ansari MA and Razdan RK 1995. Relative efficacy of various oils in repelling mosquitoes. Indian J Malariology. 32(3); 104–11.

Baratta MT et al 1998. Antimicrobial and antioxidant properties of some commercial essential oils. Flavour and Fragrance J. 13(4); 235–44.

Carlini EA et al 1986. Pharmacology of lemongrass (*Cymbopogon citratus* Stapf). J Ethnopharmacol. 17(1); 37–64.

Danlami U et al 2011. Comparative study on the Antimicrobial activities of the ethanolic extracts of Lemongrass and *Polyalthia longifolia*. J Applied Pharm Sci; 01(09):174–176.

Dubey NK et al 1997. Citral: a cytotoxic principle isolated from the essential oil of *Cymbopogon citratus* against P388 leukemia cells. Currente Sci. 73(1); 22–4.

Ferriera MSC and Fonteles MC 1985. Activity of the essential oil of *Cymbopogon citratus* on sleeping time in rats. Brazilian J Med Biol Res. 18(5/6); A 724.

Figueirinha A et al 2010. Anti-Inflammatory Activity of *Cymbopogon citratus* Leaf infusion in Lipopoly saccharide-Stimulated Dendritic Cells: Contribution of the Polyphenols. J Med Food; 13(3):681–690.

Garg D et al 2012. Comparative Analysis of Phytochemical Profile and Antioxidant Activity of Some Indian Culinary

Herbs. Research Journal of Pharmaceutical, Biological and Chemical Sciences; 3(3):845–854.

Guenther E. The essential oils. New York: Van Nostrand Company, 1950.

Ibrahim D 1992. Antimicrobial activity of the essential oil of local serai, *Cymbopogon citratus*. J Biosci Bioengin. 3, (1/2),; 87–90.

Kauderer B et al 1991. Evaluation of the mutagenicity of â-myrcene in mammalian cells *in vitro*. Environ Molec Mutagenesis. 18(1); 28–34.

Moron Rodriguez F 1996. Ausencia de efectos antiinflamatorio y analgesico del extracto fluido de *Cymbopogon citratus* al 30 porciento por via oral. Revista de Plantas Medicinales. 1(2); 3–6.

Murakami A et al 1994. Possible anti-tumour promoting properties of traditional Thai food items and some of their active constituents. Asia Pacific J Clin Nutr. 3(4); 185–91.

Onabanjo AO et al 1993. Effects of aqueous extracts of *Cymbopogon citratus* in malaria. J Protozoo Res. 3(2); 40–5.

Pedroso RB et al 2006. Biological Activities of Essential Oil Obtained from Cymbopogon citrates on Crithidia deanei. Acta Protozool 2006; 45:231–240.

Rao VS et al 1990. Effect of myrcene on nociception in mice. J Pharmacy and Pharmacol. 42; 877–88.

Seth G et al 1976. Effect of essential oil of *Cymbopogon citratus* Stapf on Central Nervous- System. Ind J Exp Biol 14(3); 370–1.

Silva CdeB et al 2008. Antifungal activity of the lemongrass oil and citral against Candida spp. Braz J Infect Dis; 12(1).

Suaeyun R et al 1997. Inhibitory effects of lemon grass (*Cymbopogon citratus* Stapf) on formation of azoxymethane-induced DNA adducts and aberrant crypt foci in the rat colon. Carcinogen. 18 (5); 949- 55.

Syed M et al 1995. Essential oils of the family Gramineae with antibacterial activity. Part 2. The antibacterial activity of a local variety of *Cymbopogon citratus* oil and its dependence on the duration of storage. Pakistan J Sci Ind Res. 8(3/4); 146–8.

Tangpu V and Yadav AK 2006. Antidiarrhoeal activity of *Cymbopogon* citrates and its main constituent, citral. Pharmacologyonline; 2:290–298.

Tchoumbougnang F, et al 2005. *In vivo* antimalarial activity of essential oils from *Cymbopogon citratus* and *Ocimum gratissimum* on mice infected with *Plasmodium berghei.* Planta Med; 71(1):20–3.

Viana GSB et al 2000. Antinociceptive effect of the essential oil from *Cymbopogon citratus* in mice. J Ethnopharmacol; 70(3):323–327.

Vinitketkumnuen U et al 1994. Antimutagenicity of lemon grass (*Cymbopogon citratus*, Stapf) to various known mutagens in salmonella mutation assay. Mutat Res; 341(1):71–5.

Zheng GQ et al 1993. Potential anti-carcinogenic natural products isolated from lemongrass oil and galanga root oil. J Agric Food Chem. 41(2); 153–6.

Chapter 6 Lignum vitae *Guaiacum officinale*

Drawing of Guaiacum by Köhler-s: Medizinal-Pflanzen-069. Article from Wikipedia,

Ahmad VU et al 2004. Triterpenoid saponin from the bark of *Guaiacum officinale* L. Nat Prod Res 18(2).

Bahada-Sing PS et al 2014. Wound healing potential of *Tillandsia recurvata* and *Guaiacum officinale* in streptozotocin induced type 1 diabetic rats. Am J Biomed Life. 2(6): 146–149.

Barton MK 2014. Faecal occult blood testing remains a valuable screening tool. CA Cancer J Clin; 64: 3–4.

Dunant S 2013. Blood and Beauty. Virago.

Duwiejua M et al 1994. Anti-inflammatory Activity of *Polygonum bistorta, Guaiacum officinale* and *Hamamelis virginiana* in Rats. J Pharm and Pharmacol. 46(4); 286–290.

Eppenberger P et al 2118. A brief pictorial and historical introduction to guaiacum-from a putative cure for syphilis to an actual screening method for colorectal cancer. Br J Clin Pharmacol. 83; 2118–2119.

Fisch ME 1945, Nicolaus Pol Doctor 1494, Bulletin of the History of Medicine, 20(2): 294–298.

Fornaciari A et al 2020. Syphilis in Maria Salviati (1499–1543), wife of Giovanni de' Medici of the Black Bands. Emerg Infect Dis; 26(6):1274–1282.

Gaenger S 2015. World trade in medicinal plants from Spanish America, 1717–1815. Med Hist; 59; 44–62.

Ibrahim S et al 2018. Antidiabetic effect of *Guaiacum officinale*; on exocrine function and histopathology of pancreas in streptozocin induced diabetic rats. Prof Med J 25(4); 620–626.

Lowe HIC et al 2014. Anti HIV-1 activity of the crude extracts of *Guaiacum officinale* L (Sygophyllaceae.) Europ J Med Plants 4(4): 483–489.

Maneechai S and Pikulthong V 2017. Total phenolic contents and free radical scavenging activity of *Guaiacum officinale* L. extracts. Pharmacogn J., 9(6): 929–931.

Offiah NV and Ezenwaka CE 2003. Anti-fertility Properties of the Hot Aqueous Extract of *Guaiacum officinale*. Pharmaceutical biology. Taylor & Francis. 454–457.

Renaissance Invention: Stradanus's Nova Reperta, edited by Lia Markey, Northwestern University Press, 2020. A thorough discussion of the engraving, *Hyacum et Lues Venerea*, can be found in Chapter 6, "A New World Disease and Therapy", by Alessandra Foscati and Lia Markey.

Shoukat et al 2021. Physicochemical screening; identification of anticancer, antibacterial and antioxidant principles by fractionation and GC-MS profiling of fruits of Guaiacum officinale L. Pakistan J Sci. 73(1);13–13.

Chapter 7 Liquorice *Glycyrrhiza glabra*

Drawing of *Glycyrrhiza glabra* from a coloured lithograph after MA Burnett, c. 1847.

Acharya SK et al 1993. A preliminary open trial on interferon stimulator (SNMC) derived from *Glycyrrhiza glabra* in the treatment of subacute hepatic failure. Indian J Med Res 98:6974.

Akamatsu H et al 1991. Mechanism of anti- inflammatory action of glycyrrhizin: effect on neutrophil functions including reactive oxygen species generation. Planta Med; 57:119-121.

Arase Y et al 1997. The long term efficacy of glycyrrhizin in chronic hepatitis C patients. Cancer 79(8):1494–1500.

Bradley PR ed 1992. British Herbal Compendium, Vol. 1. Bournemouth: British Herbal Medicine Association.

Bruneton, J. 1995. Pharmacognosy, Phytochemistry, Medicinal Plants. Paris: Lavoisier Publishing.

Chang HM and But PPH eds 1986. Pharmacology and Applications of Chinese Materia Medica, Vol. 1. Philadelphia: World Scientific. 304–316.

Der Marderosian A ed 1999. The Review of Natural Products. St. Louis: Facts and Comparisons.

Foster S and Tyler VE 1999. Tyler's Honest Herbal: A Sensible Guide to the Use of Herbs and Related Remedies. New York: Haworth Herbal Press. 241243.

Foster S and Yue C 1992. Herbal Emissaries Bringing Chinese Herbs to the West. Rochester, VT: Healing Arts Press. 112121.

Indian Pharmacopoeia, Vol. 1. (IP). 1996. Delhi: Government of India Ministry of Health and Family Welfare Controller of Publications. 440442.

Karnick CR 1994. Pharmacopoeial Standards of Herbal Plants. 12. Delhi: Sri Satguru Pubs. Vol 1:158159; Vol. 2:86.

Kaur R et al 2013. Glycyrrhiza glabra: A Phytopharmacological Review. Int J Pharm Sci Res; 4(7); 2470- 2477.

Mori K et al 1990. Effects of glycyrrhizin (SNMC: stronger neo-
minophagen C) in hemophilia patients with HIV-1 infection.
Tohoku J Exp Med 162(2):183–193.

Nagai T et al 1991. The protective effect of glycyrrhizin against
injury of the liver caused by ischemia-reperfusion. Arch
Environ Contam Toxicol; 20:432-436.

Numazaki K et al 1994. Effect of glycyrrhizin in children with
liver dysfunction associated with cytomegalovirus infection.
Tohoku J Exper Med; 172:147- 153.

Pompei R., Flore O., Marccialis MA. Glycyrrhizic acid inhibits
virus growth and inactivates virus particles. Nature 1979;
281: 689-690.

Tu G ed 1992. Pharmacopoeia of the People's Republic of China,
English Edition. Beijing: Guangdong Science and Technology
Press. 118119.

Van Rossum TG et al 1999. Intravenous glycyrrhizin for
the treatment of chronic hepatitis C: a double- blind,
randomized, placebo-controlled phase I/II trial. Journal of
Gastroenterology & Hepatology; 14:1093-1099.

Wang ZY and Nixon DW 2001. Licorice and cancer. Nutr Cancer;
39:1-11.

Chapter 8 Nutmeg *Myristica fragrans*

Drawing of nutmeg from the William Farquhar Collection,
1819–1823).jpg.

Academia website, Herbal Medicine for Insomnia, Yarnell, Eric,
Alternative and Complimentary Therapies Journal, 2015,
21(4): 173–179, PDF accessed from: https://www.academia.
edu/22236184/ Herbal_medicine_for_insomnia

American Botanical Council website, HerbClipTM Online,
Tisserand, Robert, Aromatherapy as Mind-Body Medicine,
International Journal of Aromatherapy. Vol. 6, No. 3:14–19,
accessed from: http://cms.herbalgram.org/herbclip/098/
review41932.html

Ashokkumar K et al 2022. Compositional variation in the leaf, mace, kernel, and seed essential oil of nutmeg (*Myristica fragrans* Houtt) from the Western Ghats, India. Natural Product Research, 36(1), 432- 435.

Atta-ur-Rahman et al 2000. Antifungal activities and essential oil constituents of some spices from Pakistan. J Chem Soc Pakistan, 22, 60- 65.

Balick MJ and Paul AC 2000. Plants that heal people: culture of science of ethnobotany. Scientific American Library, New York.

Battaglia S 2018. The Complete Guide to Aromatherapy, 3rd Edition, Vol 1 Foundations and Materia Medica, Australia: Black Pepper Creative Pty Ltd, p. 437.

Bounatirou S 2007. Chemical composition, antioxidant and antibacterial activities of the essential oils isolated from Tunisian *Thymus capitatus* Hoff. et Link. Food chemistry. 105(1): 146–155.

Calliste C et al 2010. A new antioxidant from wild nutmeg. Food chemistry. 118(3): 489–496.

Checker R et al 2008. Immuno-modulatory and radio-protective effects of lignans derived from fresh nutmeg mace (*Myristica fragrans*) in mammalian splenocytes. Internat Immunopharmacol. 8(5): 661–669.

Chevallier A 2016. Encyclopedia of Herbal Medicine 3rd Edition, US: DK Publishing. 115.

Cho JY et al 2007. Isolation and anti-fungal activity of lignans from *Myristica fragrans* against various plant pathogenic fungi. Pest Management Sci: formerly Pesticide Science. 63(9): 935–940.

Dorman H and Deans S 2000. Antimicrobial agents from plants: antibacterial activity of plant volatile oils. J Applied Microbiol. 88(2): 308- 316.

Dorman HD and Deans SG 2004. Chemical composition, antimicrobial and in vitro antioxidant properties of *Monarda citriodora var. citriodora, Myristica fragrans, Origanum vulgare ssp. hirtum, Pelargonium sp.* and *Thymus zygis* oils. J Essential Oil Res. 16(2): 145–150.

Ellen R 1993. On the edge of the Banda zone: past and present in the social organisation of a Moluccan trading network. Honolulu: University of Hawai'i Press.

Francis SK et al 2019. Phytochemical investigation on *Myristica fragrans* stems, bark. Natural Product Research, 33, 1204–1208.

Gils CV and Cox PA 1994. Ethnobotany of nutmeg in the Spice Islands. J Ethnopharmacol. 42, 117- 124.

Gupta AD and Rajpurohit D 2011. Antioxidant and Antimicrobial Activity of Nutmeg (*Myristica fragrans*). In Nuts and Seeds in Health and Disease Prevention, Elsevier; 831–839.

Hussain S and Rao A 1991. Chemopreventive action of mace (*Myristica fragrans*, Houtt) on methylcholanthrene-induced carcinogenesis in the uterine cervix in mice. Cancer lett. 56(3): 231- 234.

Kyriakis JM et al 1994. The stress-activated protein kinase subfamily of c-Jun kinases. Nature. 369(6476): 156–160.

Malik T et al 2022. Nutmeg nutraceutical constituents: *In vitro* and *in vivo* pharmacological potential. J Food Processing and Preservation. 46(6); e15848.

Mueller M et al 2010. Anti-inflammatory activity of extracts from fruits, herbs and spices. Food Chem. 122(4): 987- 996.

Naeem N et al 2016. Nutmeg: A review on uses and biological properties. IJCBS, 9:107–110.

Nguyen PH et al 2010. AMP-activated protein kinase (AMPK) activators from *Myristica fragrans* (nutmeg) and their anti-obesity effect. Bio-organic & medicinal chemistry letters. 20(14): 4128–4131.

Olajide OA et al 2000. Evaluation of the pharmacological properties of nutmeg oil in rats and mice. Pharmaceutical biology. 38(5): 385–390.

Sabulal B et al 2006. Caryophyllene-rich rhizome oil of Zingiber nimmonii from South India: chemical characterization and antimicrobial activity. Phytochem. 67(22): 2469–2473.

Samaranyake GVP et al 2019. Efficacy of Nutmeg as a face cream on mukhadushika. Int J Sci Res Pub 09(2); 451–454.

Shetty et al 2019. Rinse Smart: Nutmeg mouthwash. JIDA 13(2); 20–24.

Taylor and Francis Online Website, Nutmeg oil alleviates chronic inflammatory pain through inhibition of COX-2 expression and substance P release in vivo, Zhang WK et al 2016. Food and Nutrition Res J, 60(1); accessed from: https://www.tandfonline.com/doi/full/10.3402/fnr.v60.30849

Tisserand R and Young R 2014. Essential Oil Safety 2nd Edition, UK: Churchill Livingstone Elsevier. 366–367.

UCLA website, Spices, Exotic Flavors and Medicines, Nutmeg and Mace, accessed from: https://unitproj.library.ucla.edu/biomed/spice/ index.cfm?displayID=19

Ultee A et al 2002. The phenolic hydroxyl group of carvacrol is essential for action against the food-borne pathogen *Bacillus cereus*. Applied Environ Microbiol. 68(4): 1561–1568.

Vasantrao Padol M et al 2022. Comparative evaluation of nutmeg mouthwash and 0.2% chlorhexidine gluconate mouthwash on halitosis and plaque control: A randomized clinical trial. J Indian Soc Periodontal 26(4); 384–389.

Chapter 9 Senna *Cassia angustifolia, Cassia senna (syn. Cassia acutifolia, Senna alexandrina)*

Drawing of senna: Tab. 80 from Vervolg ob de Avbeeldingen der artseny-gewassen met derzelver Nederduitsche en Latynsche beschryvingen, Eersde Deel from Kurt Stüber 1813 http://www.biolib.de

Aboelsoud NH 2010. Herbal medicine in ancient Egypt. J Med Plant Res; 4(2):82–86.

Blumenthal M et al eds 1998.The Complete German Commission E Monographs - Therapeutic Guide to Herbal Medicines. Austin, TX: American Botanical Council; Boston, MA: Integrative Medicine Communication.

Brinckmann J and Smith T. Senna. *Cassia angustifolia* and *Cassia senna* (syn *Cassia acutifolia, Senna alexandrina*) Family: Fabaceae (Leguminosae.) Herbalgram 120; 6–13.

Ewe K et al 1993. Influence of senna, fibre, and fibre + senna on colonic transit in loperamide-induced constipation. Pharmacology; 47(Suppl. 1): 242–248.

Flückiger FA and Hanbury D 1874. Pharmacographia a History of the Principal Drugs of Vegetable Origin, met with in Great Britain and British India. London, UK: Macmillan and Co.

Greenhalf JO and Leonard HS 1973. Laxatives in the treatment of constipation in pregnant and breast-feeding mothers. *Practitioner*; 210(256): 259–263.

Linné Cv, Salvius L. Caroli Linnaei... Species plantarum: exhibentes plantas rite cognitas, ad genera relatas, cum differentiis specificis, nominibus trivialibus, synonymis selectis, locis natalibus, secundum systema sexuale digestas... Holmiae (Stockholm, Sweden): Impensis Laurentii Salvii; 1753.

McGovern PE et al 2009. Ancient Egyptian herbal wines. Proc Natl Acad Sci USA; 106(18): 7361–7366.

Nesbitt M let al 2010. Linking biodiversity, food and nutrition: The importance of plant identification and nomenclature. J Food Compos Anal; 23(6):486–498.

Radaelli F et al 2005. High-dose senna compared with conventional PEG-ES lavage as bowel preparation for elective colonoscopy: a prospective, randomized, investigator-blinded trial. Am J Gastroenterol; 100: 2674.

Ramkumar D and Rao SSC 2005. Efficacy and safety of traditional medical therapies for chronic constipation: systematic review. Am J Gastroenterol; 100(4): 936–971.

Shelton MG 1980. Standardized senna in the management of constipation in the puerperium - a clinical trial. S Afr Med J; 57(3):78–80.

Ulbricht C et al 2011. An evidence-based systematic review of senna (*Cassia senna*) by the Natural Standard Research Collaboration. J Diet Suppl; 8(2):189–238.

US Food and Drug Administration 1975. Proposal To Establish Monographs for OTC Laxative, Antidiarrheal, Emetic, and Antiemetic Products. Federal Register; 40(56):12902–12944.

Valverde A et al 1999. Senna vs polyethylene glycol for mechanical preparation the evening before elective colonic or rectal resection: A multicenter controlled trial. Arch Surg; 134(5): 514–519.

Warmington EH 1928. Commerce Between the Roman Empire and India. Cambridge, UK: Cambridge University Press.

Wendrich WZ et al 2003. Berenike crossroads: the integration of information. J Econ Soc Historie; 46(1):46–87.

Wood GB and Bache F 1833. The Dispensatory of the United States of America. Philadelphia, PA: Grigg & Elliot.

Part 4 Poisonous Plants in Renaissance Florence

Aakhus P 2008. Astral Magic in the Renaissance: Gems, Poetry, and Patronage of Lorenzo de' Medici. 3(2): 185–206.

Al-Snafi AE 2017. Medical importance of *Datura fastuosa* (syn: *Datura metel*) and *Datura stramonium* - A review. IOSR Journal Of Pharmacy. 7(2) Version. 1 43–58.

Bacci A 1573. L'alicorno, Florence. Giorgio Marescotti.

Bacci A 1587. Le XII pietre pretiose, le quali per ordine di Dio nella Santa Legge, adornano I vestimenti del sommo Sacerdote. Aggiuntevi il diamante, le margarite, e l'oro poste da S. Giovanni nell'Apocalisse in figura della celeste Gerusalemme: con un sommario dell'altre pietre pretiose, Rome, Bartolomeo Grassi.

Barker S 2008. The art of poison. The Florentine.

Barker S 2017. Poisons and the Prince: Toxicology and Statecraft at the Medici Grand Ducal Court. Chap 7; 71–82. in Toxicology in the Middle Ages and Renaissance. History of toxicology and environmental health. The Medici Archive Project, Florence Italy.

Cassar P 1987. An outline history of pharmacy: part 2: Renaissance to twentieth century. https://www.um.edu.mt/library/oar/handle/123456789/48257

Chan TY 2012. Aconite poisoning following the percutaneous absorption of *Aconitum* alkaloids. Forensic Sci. Int. 223, 25–27.

Codronchi GB 1595. De morbis veneficis ac veneficiis (On Poisoning Diseases and Poisoners.)

Cooper MR and Johnson AW 1984. Poisonous Plants in Britain and other effects on Animals and Man. Ministry of Agriculture, Fisheries Food, 161: 219–220.

Dioscorides: Materia Medica. Codex Vindobonensis Aniciae Julianae 512 CE.

Dutta UC 1980. Materia Medica of Hindus. 3rd edn. Varanasi. Krishnadas Academy. 2. 200p

Fisher-Homberger E 1980. Gift und Zauber, Mediziner und Apotheker. Schweizerische Ärtzezeitung 61.51: 3399–3406.

Fornaciari G 2006. The mystery of beard hairs. BMJ; 333:1299.

Gabrani G 2012. Antiproliferative Effect of *Solanum nigrum* on Human Leukemic Cell Lines. Indian J Pharm Sci; 74(5): 451–453.

Grieves M 1931. A Modern Herbal.

Guo R 2018. Botany, Phytochemistry, Pharmacology and Toxicity of *Strychnos nux-vomica* L.: A Review. Am J Chinese Med 46(01); 1–23.

Haux 1999. Digitoxin is a potential anticancer agent for several types of cancer. Med Hypotheses 53(6); 543–548.

Hibbert C 1998. The Rise and Fall of the House of the Medici's. London: The Folio Society, 1998.

JA Klocke 1989. Plant compounds as source and models of insect-control agents. In Economic and medicinal plant research. Vol 3. Ed Wagner H, Farnsworth NR and Hikino H. Academic Press NY, London.

Justice KK et al 2012. A Textbook of Medical Jurisprudence and Toxicology, 24th edn. Lexis Nexis Nagpur, chap 11; 241- 244

Kawalekar JS et al 2012. Preliminary Phytochemical Investigations on Roots of Nerium Oleander, Linn. Int J Pharmacog Phytochem Res. 4(3); 134–138.

Knott J 2014. Aconite ("Wolf's bane"; "Leopard's bane"; "Women's bane"; "Venus's Chariot"; "Scorpion"; "Monkshood;" "Blue Rocket"), "Queen-Mother" of Poisons: its place in History, in Mythology, in Criminology; in Botany, in Therapeutics, and in Toxicology. Dublin J Med Sci (1872–1920) 123; 300–308. (1907).

Magnificenza alla Corte dei Medici 1997. Electa, Milan

Mari F 2006.The mysterious death of Francesco I de' Medici and Bianca Cappello: an arsenic murder? BMJ; 23; 333(7582): 1299–1301.

Mercati M 1576. Istruttione sopra i veleni [5 Istruttione sopra la peste di Michele Mercati. . .aggiuntevi tre altre instruttioni: Sopra i veleni occultamente ministrati, Podagra & Paralisi], Rome, Vincentio Accolto.

Ms, BNCF, Magl. XXV, 18.

Mulvey-Roberts M 2012. The Encyclopedia of the Gothic. Wiley Online Library.

Perger, von K. Ritter. 1864. Deutsche Pflanzensagen. Stuttgart and Oehringen: Schaber.

Rankin A 2021. The Poison Trials. Wonder drugs, experiment and the battle for authority in Renaissance Science. Uni Chicago Press.

Retief FP and Cilliers L. Poisoning during the Renaissance: The Medicis and the Borgias

Scot R 1584. Discoverie of Witchcraft.

Shakespeare W. Hamlet, I.v.61.

Shakespeare W. Antony and Cleopatra, I.v.2,4.

Thorndike L 1934. A history of magic and experimental sciences, Vol. IV, New York, Columbia University Press.

Wexler P ed. Toxicology in the Middle Ages and Renaissance.

Williams EC 2009. Pharmacognosy. 16th edn. Elsevier Limited.

Williams DG 2013. Larvicidal potential of the leaf extract of *Datura stramonium* and *Occimum gratissimum* against *Culex quinquefasciatus* mosquito species. MSc thesis, Faculty of Science, Amadu Bello University- Zaria 2013.

MOON BOOKS
PAGANISM & SHAMANISM

What is Paganism? A religion, a spirituality, an alternative belief system, nature worship? You can find support for all these definitions (and many more) in dictionaries, encyclopaedias, and text books of religion, but subscribe to any one and the truth will evade you. Above all Paganism is a creative pursuit, an encounter with reality, an exploration of meaning and an expression of the soul. Druids, Heathens, Wiccans and others, all contribute their insights and literary riches to the Pagan tradition. Moon Books invites you to begin or to deepen your own encounter, right here, right now.

If you have enjoyed this book, why not tell other readers by posting a review on your preferred book site.

Readers of ebooks can buy or view any of these bestsellers by clicking on the live link in the title. Most titles are published in paperback and as an ebook. Paperbacks are available in traditional bookshops. Both print and ebook formats are available online.

Find more titles and sign up to our readers' newsletter
www.collectiveinkbooks.com/paganism

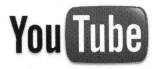

For video content, author interviews and more, please subscribe to our YouTube channel.

MoonBooksPublishing

Follow us on social media for book news, promotions and more:

Facebook: Moon Books

Instagram: @MoonBooksCI

X: @MoonBooksCI

TikTok: @MoonBooksCI